Water Learning

Susan J. Grosse, MS

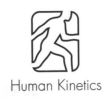

Human Kinetics

Library of Congress Cataloging-in-Publication Data

Grosse, Susan J., 1946-
   Water learning / Susan J. Grosse.
      p. cm.
   Includes bibliographical references.
   ISBN-13: 978-0-7360-6766-9 (soft cover)
   ISBN-10: 0-7360-6766-3 (soft cover)
   1. Aquatic exercises. 2. Physical education for children. 3. Motor ability in
children. I. Title.
   GV838.53.E94G76 2007
   613.7'16--dc22

                                                                2007001999

ISBN-10: 0-7360-6766-3
ISBN-13: 978-0-7360-6766-9

The Web addresses cited in this text were current as of March 29, 2007, unless otherwise noted.

Acquisitions Editor: Jill E. White; **Managing Editor:** Bethany J. Bentley; **Assistant Editor:** Anne Rumery; **Copyeditor:** Annette Pierce; **Proofreader:** Erin Cler; **Graphic Designer:** Nancy Rasmus; **Graphic Artist:** Dawn Sills; **Cover Designer:** Keith Blomberg; **Photographer (interior and cover):** Neil Bernstein, unless otherwise noted; **Photo Office Assistant:** Jason Allen; **Printer:** United Graphics

We thank the F.J. Gaenslen School in Milwaukee, Wisconsin for assistance in providing the location for the photo shoot for this book.

Human Kinetics books are available at special discounts for bulk purchase. Special editions or book excerpts can also be created to specification. For details, contact the Special Sales Manager at Human Kinetics.

Printed in the United States of America   10 9 8 7 6 5 4 3 2 1

Human Kinetics
Web site: www.HumanKinetics.com

United States: Human Kinetics
P.O. Box 5076
Champaign, IL 61825-5076
800-747-4457
e-mail: humank@hkusa.com

Canada: Human Kinetics
475 Devonshire Road Unit 100
Windsor, ON N8Y 2L5
800-465-7301 (in Canada only)
e-mail: orders@hkcanada.com

Europe: Human Kinetics
107 Bradford Road
Stanningley
Leeds LS28 6AT, United Kingdom
+44 (0) 113 255 5665
e-mail: hk@hkeurope.com

Australia: Human Kinetics
57A Price Avenue
Lower Mitcham, South Australia 5062
08 8372 0999
e-mail: liaw@hkaustralia.com

New Zealand: Human Kinetics
Division of Sports Distributors NZ Ltd.
P.O. Box 300 226 Albany
North Shore City
Auckland
0064 9 448 1207
e-mail: info@humankinetics.co.nz

contents

activity finder   v
foreword   xvii
preface   xix
acknowledgments   xxi

part I   Foundations of Water Learning

chapter 1   Introducing Children to Water Learning   3

chapter 2   Implementing Water Learning   19

chapter 3   Considering Health and Safety   27

part II   Water Learning Activities

chapter 4   Water Learning Activities for the
            Nonpool Environment   37

chapter 5   Water Learning Activities for the
            Pool Environment   91

chapter 6   Planning and Assessment   149

resources   167
about the author   170

activity finder

Learning Reinforced

Use this section of the activity finder to locate activities that reinforce specific learning and motor development concepts.

Learning reinforced	Activity names	Page numbers
Auditory perception	Be a Star	130
	Musical Spots	131
	Safe Spot	129
Balance	Advanced Balance Board	145
	Balance Board	142
	Be a Star	130
	Boat Crawl	94
	Boat Statue	95
	Bouncy Chute	122
	Chute Balance	125
	Enhanced Movement Exploration	112
	Free Ride	126
	Noodle Balance	115
	Noodle Balance Beam	119
	Noodle Locomotion	120
	On the Spot	132
	Poly Trail	133
	Statue	136
	Step Trail	137
	Tippy Board	144
	Wet Dressing	96
	Wonderboard Aerobics	146
	Wonderboard Spud	148
Big and little	Big and Little	39
Blowing	Blow	41
	Face Dunks and Bubbles	50
	Face Dunks and Counting	51
	Water Soap Bubbles	86

(continued)

(continued)

Learning reinforced	Activity names	Page numbers
Body awareness	Body Painting	42
	Dry Brush Body Painting	48
	Sprinkle	75
	Water Body Painting	84
Body image	Advanced Balance Board	145
	Balance Board	142
	Boat Crawl	94
	Boat Statue	95
	Cleanup	46
	Enhanced Movement Exploration	112
	Noodle Balance	115
	Noodle Balance Beam	119
	On the Spot	132
	Tippy Board	144
	Wash Me	140
	Washcloth Fitness	139
	Wet Dressing	96
	Where Am I?	141
	Wonderboard Aerobics	146
Body-part identification	Body Painting	42
	Dry Brush Body Painting	48
	Hand and Foot Prints	58
	Soap Up	65
	Sponge Fight	73
	Sponge Off	74
	Squirt Your Body	79
	Water Body Painting	84
Breath control	Blow	41
	Face Dunks	49
	Face Dunks and Bubbles	50
	Face Dunks and Counting	51
	Higher and Higher, Lower and Lower	118
	Picture Identification	62
	Water Soap Bubbles	86
	Water Talking	87
Capacity	Carton Pour	45
	Full and Empty	55
	Size and Shape	70
	Squirt and Fill	77
Cardiorespiratory fitness	Enhanced Movement Exploration	112
	Lion Hunt	103
	Movement Basics	110
	Noodle Balance	115
	Parachute Aerobics	121
	Step Aerobics	138
	Washcloth Fitness	139
	Wonderboard Aerobics	146

Learning reinforced	Activity names	Page numbers
Cleanup	Cleanup	46
	Paint Mix	60
	Shape Cleanup	67
Color recognition	Body Painting	42
	Bristle Blocks	44
	Color Match	106
	Color Bucket Sort	47
	Color Object Sort	93
	Noodle Structures	116
	Paint Mix	60
	Pick Up Chips	61
Counting	Bristle Blocks	44
	Circuit Training	98
	Count, Add, and Subtract	109
	Face Dunks and Counting	51
	Pick Up Chips	61
	Spot Tag	134
Creativity	Be a Star	130
	Enhanced Movement Exploration	112
	Interpretive Movement	101
	Lion Hunt	103
	Movement Basics	110
	Musical Activities	114
	Statue	136
Daily living activities	Body Painting	42
	Cleanup	46
	Hair Wash	56
	Paint Mix	60
	Shape Cleanup	67
	Soap Up	65
	Sprinkle	75
	Wash Me	140
	Wet Dressing	96
Dance	Musical Activities	114
Directionality	Enhanced Movement Exploration	112
	Higher and Higher, Lower and Lower	118
	Lion Hunt	103
	Movement Basics	110
	Noodle Locomotion	120
	Parachute Aerobics	121
	Poly Trail	133
	Step Trail	137
	Where Am I?	141
Dressing and undressing	Wet Dressing	96

(continued)

(continued)

Learning reinforced	Activity names	Page numbers
Empty and full	Carton Pour	45
	Fill the Bucket	52
	Full and Empty	55
	Pour and Fill	63
	Scoop and Fill	66
Endurance	Enhanced Movement Exploration	112
	Lion Hunt	103
	Movement Basics	110
	Noodle Balance	115
	Noodle Locomotion	120
	Parachute Aerobics	121
	Step Aerobics	138
	Washcloth Fitness	139
	Wonderboard Aerobics	146
Eye–hand coordination	Carton Pour	45
	Hammering	57
	Oops!	123
	Pour and Fill	63
	Scoop and Fill	66
	Shape Sort	68
	Splash	71
	Sponge Catch	72
	Sponge Fight	73
	Sponge Off	74
	Squirt and Fill	77
	Squirt Guns	78
	Squirt Your Body	79
	Water Sidewalk and Wall Painting	85
	Wonderboard Spud	148
Find	Take Out	81
Finger dexterity	Big and Little	39
	Block Sort	40
	Bristle Blocks	44
	Fill the Bucket	52
	Flat and Round	54
	Ice Fishing	59
	Paint Mix	60
	Pick Up Chips	61
	Round and Square	64
	Squirt and Fill	77
	Squirt Guns	78
	Squirt Your Body	79
	Stacking	80
	Take Out	81
	Underwater Puzzles	82
	Water Sidewalk and Wall Painting	85
	Wet Dressing	96

Learning reinforced	Activity names	Page numbers
Finger strength	Block Sort	40
	Bristle Blocks	44
Fit	Block Sort	40
Flat and round	Flat and Round	54
Flexibility	Boat Crawl	94
	Boat Statue	95
	Lion Hunt	103
	Wet Dressing	96
Floating (buoyancy)	Block Sort	40
	Sink or Float?	107
	Sink the Blocks	69
	Stacking	80
Following directions	Safe Spot	129
	Statue	136
Gait training	Poly Trail	133
	Step Aerobics	138
	Step Trail	137
Grasp and release	Big and Little	39
	Block Sort	40
	Bristle Blocks	44
	Color Bucket Sort	47
	Color Match	106
	Color Object Sort	93
	Ice Fishing	59
	Paint Mix	60
	Pick Up Chips	61
	Sink or Float?	107
	Sponge Catch	72
	Sponge Fight	73
	What's What?	108
	Where Am I?	141
Grasp and squeeze	Bouncy Chute	122
	Chute Balance	125
	Fill the Bucket	52
	Free Ride	126
	Hammering	57
	Oops!	123
	Parachute Aerobics	121
	Squeeze	76
	Squirt and Fill	77
	Squirt Guns	78
	Squirt Your Body	79
	Switch	124
	Wring Out	89

(continued)

(continued)

Learning reinforced	Activity names	Page numbers
Hair washing	Hair Wash	56
Hammering	Hammering	57
Hand and arm strength and endurance	Bouncy Chute	122
	Carton Pour	45
	Chute Balance	125
	Cleanup	46
	Fill the Bucket	52
	Free Ride	126
	Full and Empty	55
	Hammering	57
	Oops!	123
	Pour and Fill	63
	Scoop and Fill	66
	Shape Cleanup	67
	Size and Shape	70
	Splash	71
	Sponge Catch	72
	Sponge Fight	73
	Sponge Off	74
	Squeeze	76
	Squirt and Fill	77
	Squirt Guns	78
	Squirt Your Body	79
	Switch	124
	Water Sidewalk and Wall Painting	85
	Wring Out	89
Hard and soft	Splash	71
Heavy and light	Sink the Blocks	69
	Wet and Heavy	88
Identifying food and cooking items	Find the Food	53
Imitation	Circuit Training	98
	Lion Hunt	103
	Statue	136
In and out	Noodle Structures	116
Kinesthetic awareness	Dry Brush Body Painting	48
	Wash Me	140
	Washcloth Fitness	139
	Water Body Painting	84
Laterality	Enhanced Movement Exploration	112
	Lion Hunt	103
	Parachute Aerobics	121
	Poly Trail	133

Learning reinforced	Activity names	Page numbers
	Shape Sort	68
	Step Trail	137
	Where Am I?	141
Letter recognition	Alphabet Spots	128
	Shape Cleanup	67
Locomotion in water	Movement Basics	110
Matching	Color Bucket Sort	47
	Color Match	106
	Color Object Sort	93
	Cone Matching	99
	Count, Add, and Subtract	109
	Find the Food	53
	Shape Sort	68
	Sink or Float?	107
	What's What?	108
Math	Alphabet Spots	128
	Cone Math	100
	Count, Add, and Subtract	109
	Pick Up Chips	61
Memory	Picture Identification	62
	Switch	124
Motor control	Musical Spots	131
Motor planning	Boat Crawl	94
Number recognition	Alphabet Spots	128
	Cone Math	100
	Switch	124
Object identification	Find the Food	53
	Picture Identification	62
	Take Out	81
	What's What?	108
Object permanence	Underwater Puzzles	82
Object retrieval	Color Match	106
	Cone Matching	99
	Sink or Float?	107
Over and under	Noodle Structures	116
Physical fitness	Circuit Training	98
Printing	Water Sidewalk and Wall Painting	85
Reading signs	Circuit Training	98
Round and square	Round and Square	64
	Shape Sort	68

(continued)

(continued)

Learning reinforced	Activity names	Page numbers
Safety	Safe Spot	129
	Tippy Board	144
	Wash Me	140
Shape discrimination	Block Sort	40
	Size and Shape	70
Shape matching	Block Sort	40
Shape recognition	Shape Cleanup	67
Showering	Sprinkle	75
Size	Stacking	80
Size discrimination	Size and Shape	70
Sorting	Color Bucket Sort	47
	Color Object Sort	93
Spatial orientation	Be a Star	130
	Enhanced Movement Exploration	112
	Higher and Higher, Lower and Lower	118
	Lion Hunt	103
	Movement Basics	110
	Noodle Locomotion	120
	Noodle Structures	116
	Poly Trail	133
	Spot Tag	134
	Switch	124
	Tippy Board	144
	Where Am I?	141
Speed, distance, and height	Movement Basics	110
Spelling	Alphabet Spots	128
	Shape Cleanup	67
Splash	Splash	71
Strength	Boat Crawl	94
	Boat Statue	95
	Noodle Balance	115
	Noodle Locomotion	120
	Parachute Aerobics	121
	Step Aerobics	138
	Washcloth Fitness	139
	Wet Dressing	96
	Wonderboard Aerobics	146
Submersion	Higher and Higher, Lower and Lower	118
	Noodle Structures	116
Take and put	Take Out	81
Temperature	Ice Fishing	59

Learning reinforced	Activity names	Page numbers
Throwing and catching	Wonderboard Spud	148
Visual discrimination	Picture Identification	62
Visual perception	Alphabet Spots Underwater Puzzles	128 82
Washing	Body Painting Cleanup Soap Up Wash Me	42 46 65 140

Equipment

Use this section of the activity finder to locate activities that use particular pieces of equipment. Using the same equipment in different ways helps facilitate the transfer of learning. In addition to the items listed here, many of the activities require a bucket of water. Specific sizes and quantities are indicated in the activity description.

Equipment	Activity names	Page numbers
Activity cards	Circuit Training	98
Alphabet shapes	Big and Little Shape Cleanup	39 67
Aqua steps	Statue Step Aerobics Step Trail	136 138 137
Balls	Boat Crawl Boat Statue Bouncy Chute Flat and Round Oops! Round and Square Wonderboard Spud	94 95 122 54 123 64 148
Big boat	Boat Crawl Boat Statue Color Object Sort	94 95 93
Blocks	Big and Little Block Sort Color Bucket Sort Color Object Sort Round and Square	39 40 47 93 64

(continued)

(continued)

Equipment	Activity names	Page numbers
Blocks *(cont'd)*	Shape Sort	68
	Sink the Blocks	69
Blow tubes	Blow	41
Bristle blocks	Bristle Blocks	44
Clothing	Wet Dressing	96
Color cards	Body Painting	42
Cones	Circuit Training	98
	Cone Matching	99
	Cone Math	100
Construction paper	Hand and Foot Prints	58
	Squirt Guns	78
Containers	Body Painting	42
	Full and Empty	55
	Pour and Fill	63
	Size and Shape	70
	Squeeze	76
	Squirt and Fill	77
Cooking set	Find the Food	53
Cups	Full and Empty	55
	Hair Wash	56
	Paint Mix	60
Dishes (plastic)	Paint Mix	60
Foam shapes	Shape Cleanup	67
	Size and Shape	70
	Wet and Heavy	88
Food (play)	Find the Food	53
Ice cubes	Ice Fishing	59
Ladles	Full and Empty	55
Math cards	Cone Math	100
Mesh bags	Color Object Sort	93
Milk cartons	Carton Pour	45
	Shape Sort	68
Music	Be a Star	130
	Musical Spots	131
Noodles	Higher and Higher, Lower and Lower	118
	Noodle Balance	115
	Noodle Balance Beam	119
	Noodle Locomotion	120
	Noodle Structures	116
Object cards	Cone Matching	99

Equipment	Activity names	Page numbers
Paint	Body Painting	42
	Cleanup	46
	Paint Mix	60
Paintbrushes	Body Painting	42
	Cleanup	46
	Dry Brush Body Painting	48
	Paint Mix	60
	Water Body Painting	84
	Water Sidewalk and Wall Painting	85
Paper	Color Match	106
Parachutes	Bouncy Chute	122
	Chute Balance	125
	Free Ride	126
	Oops!	123
	Parachute Aerobics	121
	Switch	124
Pictures	Picture Identification	62
	What's What?	108
Ping-Pong balls	Shape Sort	68
Poker chips	Big and Little	39
	Flat and Round	54
	Pick Up Chips	61
Poly shapes	Alphabet Spots	128
	Be a Star	130
	Musical Spots	131
	On the Spot	132
	Poly Trail	133
	Safe Spot	129
	Spot Tag	134
Puzzles	Underwater Puzzles	82
Saxettes (or plastic recorders)	Blow	41
Scoops	Full and Empty	55
	Scoop and Fill	66
Shape container	Block Sort	40
Shovels	Scoop and Fill	66
Soap	Shape Cleanup	67
	Soap Up	65
	Water Soap Bubbles	86

(continued)

(continued)

Equipment	Activity names	Page numbers
Sponges	Cleanup	46
	Fill the Bucket	52
	Hair Wash	56
	Sponge Catch	72
	Sponge Fight	73
	Sponge Off	74
	Wet and Heavy	88
Squeeze bottles	Squeeze	76
	Squirt and Fill	77
Squirt guns	Squirt and Fill	77
	Squirt Guns	78
	Squirt Your Body	79
Stacking toys	Stacking	80
Straws	Blow	41
	Water Soap Bubbles	86
Tea set	Find the Food	53
Tubs	Face Dunks	49
	Face Dunks and Bubbles	50
	Face Dunks and Counting	51
	Hammering	57
	Hand and Foot Prints	58
	Picture Identification	62
	Underwater Puzzles	82
	Water Talking	87
Washcloths	Cleanup	46
	Soap Up	65
	Wash Me	140
	Washcloth Fitness	139
	Washcloth Substitute	83
	Wet and Heavy	88
	Where Am I?	141
	Wring Out	89
Watering cans	Body Painting	42
	Hair Wash	56
	Soap Up	65
	Sprinkle	75
Wonderboards	Advanced Balance Board	145
	Balance Board	142
	Tippy Board	144
	Wonderboard Aerobics	146
	Wonderboard Spud	148
Workbenches	Hammering	57

foreword

In the mid-1970s, when I was in Washington writing the adapted aquatics textbook for the American Red Cross, I was confronted with a deficit in my experience with children with disabilities. Although I had spent the previous 10 years working in the water with kids with disabilities, it was *pool* water: no boats involved, and I wanted to add a chapter on boating to the book. So I called Julian Stein at American Alliance for Health, Physical Education, and Recreation (AAHPER) and asked him to recommend someone who could write such a section for me. His immediate response was to recommend Sue Grosse. Sue, then at the F.J. Gaenslen School, agreed immediately, and thus began our 30-year association and friendship. In subsequent years we would meet at various professional conferences: AAHPERD, YMCA Project Aquatics, Red Cross adapted aquatics certification workshops, Council for National Cooperation in Aquatics (CNCA), and so on. Always she made significant contributions to the task at hand, sharing her knowledge and experience freely and professionally. She has continually worked as a writer and editor, providing strong leadership in the aquatic field.

Water learning and movement exploration were new concepts to aquatics people in the United States in the '70s. Swimming instructors thought only of *swimming*, and the concept of transfer in learning was not considered. Movement exploration activities were both new and enjoyable, however, and it soon became obvious that such activities would not only enhance the aquatic program but also would provide definite benefits for all children. As a combination of psychology and physical education, it provided new ideas, challenges, and opportunities.

In *Water Learning,* Sue writes comprehensively on a subject now recognized as vital. Explaining the theory concisely and clearly, she guides the reader through the rationale for various activities and facilitates the application of that theory to activities in each area. There is emphasis on safety and fun, and activities move from simple to complex. The book explains techniques of reinforcement, describes equipment, cites equipment sources, and provides evaluation tools. The book is nearly exhaustive in its approach, yet written in a way that is easy to understand and use. It is both unique and interesting and can provide endless ideas and activities for innovative aquatics instructors and leaders.

E. Louise Priest
Consultant, Aquatics Education
American Red Cross, retired
CNCA, retired

preface

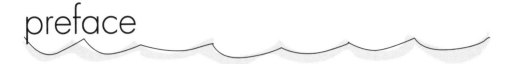

This book is for everyone who has a desire to provide good learning opportunities for children. Teachers will find new ways of reinforcing what is learned in the classroom. Physical and occupational therapists will find unique activities for accomplishing goals. Recreation personnel will find creative ideas for therapeutics as well as leisure. Parents, grandparents, and other caregivers will find ideas for supporting healthy growth and development of children.

Water learning activities can be implemented almost anywhere—schools, clinics, hospitals, homes, and community centers—because water learning does not always require the use of a swimming pool. No experience with water learning is necessary. Activities are described in detail. Additional information is provided to assist in planning water learning sessions to complement what takes place in the classroom, therapy session, or home. Equipment is relatively easy to obtain, and safety is stressed throughout.

Childhood is brief. The early childhood years are particularly important for laying the foundations of the many life processes to follow. It is important that children be provided with good learning experiences during this critical period. Play should have a purpose. Water learning is an experience whose purpose is to support and enhance learning in all other areas of a child's life.

While participating in water learning, children will develop cognition, perceptual-motor abilities, physical fitness, social interaction skills, and self-esteem. These experiences support academic development and facilitate classroom accomplishment. Water learning is designed to aid in the transfer of learning between the water environment and academic classroom, supporting achievement in math, language, science, and social studies.

Enhancing perceptual-motor abilities promotes assimilation and processing of information. Motor planning is strengthened through the development of balance, body image, laterality, directionality, and spatial orientation during water learning activities. Presented in a format based on individual decision making, water learning activities help children interact meaningfully with their environment.

Developing physical fitness not only will lead to better health but also will support and enhance acquisition of motor skills. Cardiorespiratory fitness, strength, endurance, and flexibility improve as children participate in water learning. As motor competency and physical fitness increase, so does self-esteem. Successful participation with peers, as well as interaction with facilitators, helps build social interaction skills.

What better way to learn than while having a good time? Through water learning, children find out that math is interesting. Reading and spelling become enjoyable. Viewing learning as pleasurable sets a wonderful precedent for the years of schooling to come.

Water learning activities can be integrated in all areas of a child's life. The activities can be part of physical, occupational, and recreation therapy. Water learning can be a family activity at home or at Grandma and Grandpa's house. If a pool is available, swim instructors can integrate water learning with traditional aquatics programs. Any adult can become a water learning facilitator. Information on how to implement water learning in any type of setting is provided in detail.

Chapters 1, 2, and 3 provide a thorough explanation of how to set up and lead water learning activities. Success is important in any learning process. You will learn to use a movement exploration format and a problem-solving approach to build success. Implementing water learning to support children as they grow physically and cognitively is discussed throughout. Maintaining a safe environment is important for any activity around water, so safety information is provided in detail.

Chapters 4 and 5 contain a variety of water learning activities. Each activity description includes specific information about what other learning or development the activity will reinforce. All the necessary equipment is listed. Implementation of the activity is guided by a format description with specific verbal cues and hints to generate success. An activity finder helps you select activities corresponding to the developmental and academic needs of each child.

Chapter 6 focuses on children's progress. Setting goals, planning appropriate activities, assessing and documenting results, and coordinating with other disciplines are important tasks. Coordination of these tasks is facilitated through the processes outlined here, and a water learning planning chart supports the planning process. Whether you are a teacher, therapist, parent, or swim instructor, information sharing supports the growth and development of children. Assessments are presented to make this process easy and understandable for all.

This book includes all the information you need in order to implement water learning as a worthwhile activity for any child, no matter what your experience or educational background. Regardless of learning style, experience, ability, or disability, all children can participate in and benefit from water learning activities. Water learning is easy to stage, practical, and engaging. Use this book to find out just how easy and rewarding water learning activities can be.

acknowledgments

My experiences with water learning began at F.J. Gaenslen School, in Milwaukee, Wisconsin. This was not the beginning of water learning. Water learning began with the very first water safety instructor who integrated academic concepts with preschool aquatics. I have no idea who that was. Most probably, like other wonderful educational concepts, water learning was developed by many different instructors, at many different times in history, coming to the fore when professionals recognized the broader value of the water learning concept and put information into publication.

Connie Curry Lawrence, with her movie *Splash,* and her text *Water Learning,* written with Hackett (1975), led the way. Material by Louise Priest in the American Red Cross text *Methods in Adapted Aquatics* (1976) further emphasized the value of not only water learning but also movement exploration, problem solving, and the application in aquatics of the then-emerging information on perceptual-motor development.

The water learning program at Gaenslen began in the late 1970s as a direct result of the publications of these pioneering women. Supporting optimum child growth and development while emphasizing academics, water learning activities are as important today as when I made my first discoveries. Who facilitated the discovery process? Children! It is the students of Gaenslen School you will see in our text photos.

Today's water learning program continues under the very competent direction of Carrie Paterson. Her knowledge and expertise are the foundation for the activities included here. She continues an aquatic tradition dating back to 1938 when the original Gaenslen School was built with not one but two pools. Her students, along with all our past students, have been our real instructors. They have, without exception, been willing to try activities, engage in tasks, challenge our assumed theories, and create fun out of almost anything.

Through the decades, these students, their parents, and the Gaenslen staff have been willing to share. Without this sharing, those first water learning experiences described by Lawrence, Hackett, and Priest would have remained unknown. It is a new century, and the true test of the value of a theory or practice is its survival over time. Water learning has survived and is as vital today as it was in years gone by. *Water Learning* is a testament and a thank-you to the Gaenslen family for their sharing and caring.

part I

Foundations of Water Learning

Water learning is based on the idea that interaction with water can both stimulate and enhance a child's growth and development. In the first part of the book we will investigate water learning and consider why water learning is important to a child's growth and development. You will find guidelines for establishing a safe, problem-solving learning environment.

Children grow quickly. Therefore, it is important for parents, teachers, therapists, and other caregivers to make the most of the developmental years by providing high-quality learning experiences while allowing each child to have fun and expand his or her individuality. Water learning can help make this happen for all children. In part I we will consider the following:

- What is water learning?
- How do water learning activities facilitate a child's growth and development?
- What special benefits does water learning have for children with special needs?
- How can a facilitator set up and initiate a water learning program?
- How is child safety built into water learning experiences?

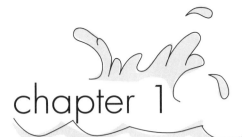

chapter 1

Introducing Children to Water Learning

Water learning refers to using water in buckets, sinks, or tubs as well as in a swimming pool or open-water setting, for educational purposes. In the early-childhood classroom, water learning activities may involve water in a sink, water table, or a collection of buckets on a waterproof surface. At home, water learning may include water in the bathtub or shower, kitchen sink, or laundry washtub. Outside, a wading pool or sprinkler may provide the water setting. If available, a shower area in a locker room is a perfect environment for water learning. In a therapy setting, the water might be in a tub on a waterproof mat, in a sink, or in several buckets on a table. A swimming pool is an obvious water learning location. You can also use a lakeshore or riverbank effectively.

Water learning uses activities in an aquatic environment to enrich and reinforce learning in nonaquatic areas of child development. Water learning is used primarily to reinforce academics. However, water learning can also reinforce motor skills, physical fitness, perceptual-motor development, and sport skills.

Adult caregivers stage water learning activities. A caregiver might be a parent or guardian, a teacher, a day-care worker, a therapist, or a recreation professional. Caregivers facilitate a child's interaction with water, which enhances the child's growth and development and supports academic growth. In this book, the term *facilitator* designates the adult that provides structure and guidance for water learning activities.

The facilitator often presents activities to the child in a questioning format—asking, rather than telling, the child to do something—and then provides whatever support might be needed for the child to successfully interact with the water environment to accomplish the task. Following completion of the initial task, the facilitator encourages the child to explore the water environment further and more creatively. This is called a *problem-solving approach* and relies heavily on movement exploration.

Because of its unique properties, water has a way of commanding and holding a child's attention and providing almost instant feedback as a result of the child's actions. Children seem to have a natural fascination with water, so why not capitalize on this focus? Water learning activities can improve the cognitive abilities of any preschool-age child. Learning about water as they use it to wash the body, fill a bucket, float an object, or make bubbles helps children gather data about the environment. Transferring regular academic subjects, such as math, reading, and science, into the pool helps children learn and can be fun.

Using a cup to pour, a large spoon to scoop, fingers to splash, and the mouth to blow helps a young child develop muscle control, physical fitness, and perceptual-motor abilities. Social interactions are facilitated when water activities of one child affect another. It is difficult to keep from splashing, and when splashed, a child usually will at least look to see what the cause is and might even splash back a response.

Children grow and develop at different rates. For children developing at a slower pace, perhaps because of a disability or lack of early opportunity, water learning activities can provide not only enrichment to the entire growth and development process but also strong support for therapeutic intervention, whether through physical, occupational, linguistic, or psychological therapy. Water learning is for all children, regardless of ability or functional level.

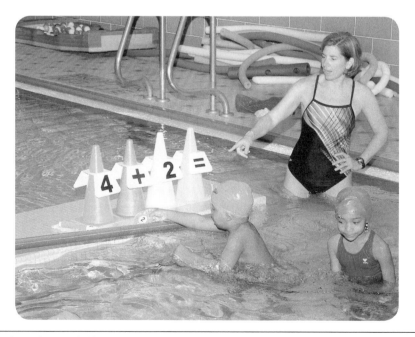

Water learning activities are not only fun, but they also can improve the cognitive abilities of preschool-age children.

More important than acquiring basic cognitive data or improving motor functioning is the child's potential for improving in two less tangible areas of development: creativity and problem solving. Programs and activities for preschool children have a definite mandate to foster creativity and cultivate development of the natural inquisitiveness of the young child. This inquisitiveness leads a child to try different solutions to problems, use tools and implements in different ways, and experiment. Children gain mastery over their environments through exploration. Water learning situations where children can directly interact with water in natural and in constructed settings can greatly affect a child's growth and development in creativity and problem solving.

Water learning does not involve learning to swim, even though activities may take place in a swimming pool. However, water learning activities can facilitate water orientation, submersion, breath holding, breath control, locomotion in water, comfort with buoyancy, balance, and ability to change direction. Water learning activities make great warm-up activities for regular swim lessons. Water learning activities also provide fun and challenging alternatives to traditional water games.

Water learning activities are not necessarily preswim activities. Although water learning can help a child become more comfortable in and around water, including submersion in water, water learning activities are a goal in and of themselves. Any contribution to learning to swim is secondary to the overriding purpose of enhancing physical, cognitive, psychological, and social growth and development.

Benefits of Water Learning

Let's take a closer look at how water learning activities can affect child growth and development. Blackmore (2003, p. 22) reminds us that "movement is an indispensable part of learning and thinking, as well as an integral part of mental processing." Water learning takes the movement component of any activity, immerses it in water, and combines it with mental processing. Water learning reinforces cognitive and perceptual-motor development. It enhances physical growth and development, as well as physical fitness. It promotes social interaction, and it facilitates emotional stability.

Because water learning involves mental activity along with physical activity, it requires thinking. Facilitators can plan activities to target specific areas of academic development or needed remediation. They can integrate basics, such as color, number, and letter recognition, along with reading, language arts, math, science, and social studies with water learning activities. Stevens-Smith (2004, p. 10) cites extensive research and concludes that "physical activity increases all-around vigor, promotes clearer thinking, and affects grade scores of children." Water learning provides this type of physical activity, thus helping children develop cognition.

Perceptual-motor abilities include the development of body image, balance, laterality, directionality, spatial orientation, and ocular pursuit (Kephart 1966). Perceptual-motor skills are not the same as cognition or intelligence. Rather, each perceptual-motor component makes its own distinct contribution to helping a child organize information about his or her world.

- Body image refers to knowing specific body parts and where they are located in relation to each other as well as their general functional contribution to exerting control over the environment.
- Balance refers to how a child controls his or her position in and movement through space while withstanding the force of gravity.
- Laterality refers to establishing an awareness of the left and right sides of the body as well as being able to move from side to side and across the body's midline.
- Directionality is the ability to move left, right, forward, backward, up, down, around, and through space, responding to the presence of other people and objects appropriately.
- Spatial orientation is the ability to move through space in any direction, responding to the presence of people and objects appropriately. It is a combination of laterality and directionality.
- Ocular pursuit refers to being able to use one's vision to track objects in space, establishing relationships among objects and people.

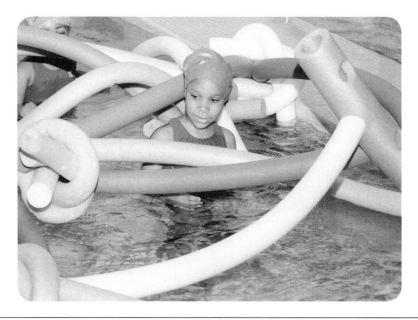

Moving around objects in the water helps children develop spatial-orientation skills.

Important for integrating sensory input with motor output, perceptual-motor activities are an integral part of early-childhood education. Mastery of perceptual-motor skills allows a child to take the sensory input from the five senses, process that input, and plan and execute motor activity in response. Combining perceptual-motor activities with water learning activities provides a multisensory approach to stimulating perceptual-motor development.

Physical growth and development are also enhanced through movement. Muscular activity stimulates circulation and respiration, critical components of cardiorespiratory fitness. As muscles respond to demands of activity, strength develops and endurance lengthens. Moving the arms and legs during activities that require the use of the large muscles of the body improves flexibility. These four areas—cardiorespiratory development, strength, endurance, and flexibility—are, along with body composition, major determiners of physical fitness.

- Cardiorespiratory fitness refers to the capacity of the heart and lungs to work together, supplying the oxygen demands of the body and contributing to development in all other body systems.
- Strength refers to the ability to sustain activity with force against resistance.
- Endurance refers to the ability to maintain activity over increasingly longer periods of time.
- Flexibility refers to the range of motion of all major joints.
- Body composition refers to how much of the body is lean mass and how much is fat.

As people develop and maintain fitness, their general health improves. For people who have difficulty moving on land, water facilitates movement. Gravity is negated because water provides support and stimulation for the body. Water learning activities are engaging. Children often forget about movement difficulties caused by obesity, inactivity, lack of experience, or a disability as they focus on water learning tasks. This means that physical growth and development can be enhanced for any child as physical fitness improves, regardless of capability or skill development.

Children find water learning activities to be fun, and they enjoy the level of success they experience. When the facilitator uses a problem-solving approach, children can choose their level of engagement and gradually increase the sophistication of their responses as their confidence increases. Praise for attempting a task, no matter what the difficulty level of the task is, increases self-esteem. Children who succeed are willing to continue trying increasingly more difficult tasks. This creates a positive engagement cycle important to emotional health. Even the most insecure child can achieve success and develop self-confidence through water learning experiences.

Social growth through play develops through many stages:

- Isolation play, with a child playing alone, starts the process.
- Two or more children engaged in isolation play, but in close proximity to each other, exemplify parallel play, the next stage in the developmental progression.
- Group interaction is the highest level of play, attained by children comfortable in their environment and comfortable with the task at hand and with each other. Often a shared task facilitates a child's progression from parallel play to group interaction. Interaction in groups of two or three children precedes interaction in large groups.

Because of the individualistic nature of the problem-solving approach, a child is allowed to participate in whatever stage of play he or she is most comfortable in. Social interaction is not required for successful experiences in water learning.

Working With Children With Disabilities

Water learning is particularly helpful in fostering the growth and development of children with disabilities. Children with cognitive disabilities need more time to learn academics. Although they may be the same chronological age as their classmates, their mental age can lag further behind as

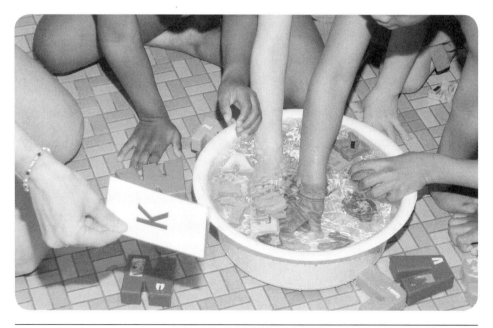

Parallel play, one of the stages of social development, takes place when children play by themselves but in close proximity to other children.

they get older. The more opportunities a child has for reinforcing what he or she learns in the classroom, the easier it will be for the child to master academics. Water learning provides for this reinforcement by transferring learning between classroom and pool.

Children with physical disabilities often have more limited opportunities for physical activities than their peers without disabilities. Time spent in hospitals and recovering from corrective surgeries precludes time spent in active play. Wearing a cast, brace, or orthotic; using a wheelchair or a walker; or contending with weak muscles or unnecessary movements are all circumstances that interfere with large-muscle activity. Water learning in a pool provides an environment that facilitates movement. Children with physical disabilities can have greater freedom of movement in water than in any other place.

Children with sensory disabilities, in many cases, need additional sensory input to compensate for the sense that is affected by disability. Water learning provides that input. Wet is a clearly defined state of being. Activities taking place in a wet environment provide unique sensory stimulation and facilitate the transfer of learning between classroom and pool, reinforcing cognitive development.

Children with psychological or neurobiological disabilities can benefit a great deal from water learning. Immersion in water demands focus of attention and awareness of reality. Some children focus in water better than anywhere else. Because the pool is, in many cases, a new environment, a child with behavioral problems will have no existing negative behaviors to rely on, making pool behavior a brand new area to develop. Children with attention-deficit/hyperactivity disorder will find an outlet for their energies and at the same time have opportunities to extend their attention span while engaged in activities to reinforce academic learning.

Social development is a concern for any child whose interactions with peers may be affected by disability. Limited opportunities for peer play, negative behaviors, lack of social skills, and underdeveloped play skills are all limiting factors. Water learning can be individual in nature, but it can also be structured to accommodate parallel play or group interaction. When water is the focus of activity, deterrents to social interaction are often less noticeable, resulting in improved social development.

Perceptual-motor disabilities often accompany other disabilities. Because children need to move in order to grow and develop, a lack of movement opportunities during early childhood may also affect perceptual-motor development. Children with problems in body image, balance, laterality (handedness), directionality, and spatial organization benefit from the problem-solving approach and the multisensory nature of water learning.

Developmental coordination disorder is characterized by clumsy, awkward motor behavior absent of a physiological cause. Relatively new to the *Diagnostic and Statistical Manual of Mental Disorders* lexicon, this disorder affects a considerable number of children, most of whom can benefit from water learning (American Psychiatric Association 1994, p. 943). A pool environment provides a safe place for children to work on locomotor skills. Water learning activities are engaging and fun. Free from the fear of falling or colliding with objects when moving on land, children in water move with greater confidence, building muscle strength and endurance and motor control.

Stein (2004, p. 21) aptly summarizes the value of integrating academic goals with aquatic therapy: "Approached in appropriate ways, aquatic therapy for physiological purposes can also become academic (brain development) therapy, with focus still on therapeutic goals and objectives, but also integrating appropriate academic concepts." This is, in effect, water learning.

Facilitating Water Learning

Water learning does not happen randomly. Simply supplying a child with equipment and a water supply does not guarantee positive results. For water learning activities to have maximum benefits for the growth and development of any child, adult structure and guidance are necessary. Using a multisensory approach, implementing a problem-solving format, following logical progressions, and maintaining a success-oriented atmosphere greatly enhance all water learning activities. Facilitating perceptual-motor development supports development in many other areas. Having a variety of quality learning activities that can be implemented almost anywhere makes water learning functional for teachers, therapists, parents, or anyone wanting to enrich a child's life.

Multisensory Approach

People learn by gathering information through their senses and then using their brain to process that information. If they see something, they are receiving information through one sense. If they see and hear something at the same time, learning is enhanced as information enters the brain through two different avenues. For example, if, while you are driving, you see a stop sign, you might stop. However, if you see the stop sign and your passenger calls out "Stop!" you are more likely to stop because your information input has doubled. Using a multisensory approach during water learning activities helps each child learn by providing input through several senses. Therefore, when implementing a water learning activity, follow these guidelines:

- Provide verbal as well as physical cues for difficult tasks. For example, when asking a child to use just one hand, also gently tap the hand to be used. Some children will benefit from hands-on assistance.

- When a child touches something, describe it. For example, when a child picks up a blue block, say, "That block is blue."
- Provide descriptive vocabulary for new or different sensations a child may be feeling, for example, "Yes, the water is wet."
- Encourage the child to say back to you what he or she is doing. For example, as the child selects the big objects from a bucket containing a variety of objects, encourage the child to repeat, "I am getting the big ones."

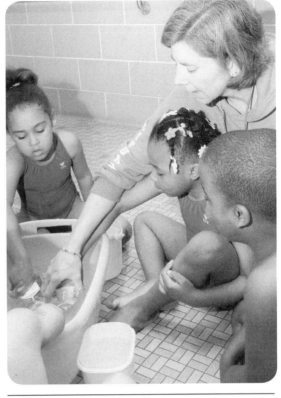

Both verbal and physical cues are helpful when teaching young children.

A multisensory approach is not advisable for every child. Some disabilities cause a child's nervous system to be hypersensitive to stimulation. A child showing discomfort or agitation during multisensory activities may be experiencing sensory overload. In such cases, adjust activities to limit sensory input, particularly input from the surrounding environment, and structure activities so that information is presented to one sense at a time.

Problem-Solving Format

Placing the child in control of decisions about engagement and task accomplishment increases his or her comfort in the activity and desire to try. Problem solving is particularly useful in fostering development because it allows children to make choices about how they will attempt and complete activities. Using a problem-solving format means structuring tasks by asking the child a question (rather than giving a direction). "Can you pick up only the red chips?" is a problem-solving question. "Pick up the red chips" is a direction.

To begin a problem-solving activity, ask the child a question beginning with "can you." Then, watch the child's response. If the response is what you had in mind when you asked the question, offer praise and proceed to the next problem. If the response is not what you intended, or if you think the child can do better, ask another, more qualifying question. The following are examples:

Goal: To have the child differentiate between movements that are fast and movements that are slow.

Activity: Moving around the pool, ask, "Can you move around our pool space?" As the child is moving, ask, "Can you move faster?" If the child's speed remains the same, ask again, emphasizing the word *faster*. If you are modeling movements, be sure you move faster. If the child answers you by saying yes or no, ask the child to show you what he or she means. Ask several "faster" questions and then switch to "Can you move very slowly?" Be sure to change the speed of your pronunciation of *slowly* to aid in cuing.

This type of problem solving allows a child to make several choices. He or she can select the type of movement used (none was specified, so walking is fine, and so is scooting around holding the pool gutter). The child can also select how fast he or she travels and in which direction and which body parts to use. For these reasons, the problem-solving approach is appropriate for children of various ability levels.

Problem solving also includes lots of praise. Because children can select their level of engagement, all honest attempts to solve a problem are worthy of praise. Engagement is what the facilitator desires. Once the child engages in the problem, it is up to the facilitator to refine subsequent problem-solving questions until he or she obtains the desired level of response. In the process, each of the child's responses is praise worthy. From an emphatic "Yes!" and "Excellent job, Johnny!" to a specific comment such as "You really can move quickly, Li, and you are still able to stop when the music stops," praise is crucial to the child's continuing engagement and accomplishment. Praise often, smile, and clap. Show the child that what he or she is doing is not just great, but fantastic.

The following are characteristics of problem-solving water learning activities:

- They are progressive, beginning with very easy tasks and gradually progressing to more complex.

- They involve large-muscle motor control, graduating to small-muscle motor coordination.

- They start with single tasks and gradually progress to a sequence of multiple tasks.

- They provide multisensory input.
- They are appropriate for the child's chronological and developmental age.
- They use existing skills and abilities to build new skills and abilities.
- They reinforce learning in at least one other area of growth and development.

The more a child responds to questions, the more the child solves problems. Children learn by solving problems. To facilitate problem solving, follow these guidelines:

- Ask questions as you begin a task. Begin with questions such as "Can you sort (or find, put, pour, empty, take, squeeze, brush, paint, wash, sprinkle, or dry)?"
- Help the child develop the quality of his or her responses by asking additional quantifying questions using words such as more, less, faster, slower, more carefully, wetter, dryer, and cleaner.
- Consider any attempt a child makes to solve the problem to be a success, even if the problem or task is not solved or completed. Praise the child and the effort, and then ask a further qualifying question. For example, after asking LaTasha, "Can you put water from this full bucket into the empty one?" she dips her hand in the water and tries to grab some water and put it into the other bucket. This doesn't result in much water being transferred and LaTasha stops. First, praise her for getting some water into the empty bucket (even a few drops). Then ask "Can you get *more* water into the empty bucket?" or "How can you get more water into the empty bucket?" or "Is there something else you can use to put water into the empty bucket?" Additional questions will help LaTasha learn how to accomplish tasks. Although giving directions might take less time, water learning activities are not time dependent. Facilitating learning by allowing the child to solve the problem is a much more important goal.
- Rephrase questions if a child's response is only a verbal "no." Asking a question provides an opportunity for a child to answer no. If this should occur, do not view this response as an issue worthy of a struggle. Rather, rephrase the question into a challenge. "Can you fill the bucket with water?" can be rephrased into the challenge "Show me how you can fill the bucket with water." Adding encouraging comments such as "I know you can do it!" and "Try" will provide support during the attempt at the challenge. Provide additional assistance with hands-on guidance during a child's initial attempt at a difficult task.

Can every child respond to questions or challenges? No. A child with a severe disability may not be able to respond independently to task questions or challenges. However, using this approach is still important, even if the facilitator must physically help the child perform the task. Asking the question or posing the challenge and then providing an answer facilitates cognitive development, even in situations where a child has a severe disability or multiple disabilities. Provide hands-on assistance until the child can make his or her response independently.

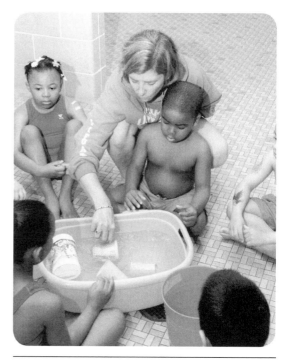

Hands-on assistance is often necessary when teaching young children.

Logical Progression

Development occurs in stages. These stages can be predictable. Learning is facilitated if tasks and activities take advantage of what is known about progressive development. In selecting tasks and activities, remember the following:

- Gross motor development occurs before fine motor development. As a result, a child is able to pick up a large object before he or she can pick up a small object.

- Gross motor development occurs from the midline of the body outward. As a result, a child is able to move the whole arm before he or she develops finger control.

- Hands can control objects on the same side of the body before they can control objects on the opposite side (across the midline). As a result, a child using the right hand has greater success manipulating something placed to the right of center of the body than something placed on the left.

- Eye–hand coordination develops for stationary objects before it develops for moving objects.

- Ability to follow one-part directions comes before the ability to follow two-part sequences. Following two-part sequences comes before following three-part sequences, and so forth. Therefore, start with single-solution problems, and gradually make tasks more complex.

- The tasks should progress from known to unknown, simple to complex, and easy to difficult.

Perceptual-Motor Integration

Development of body image, balance, laterality, directionality, spatial orientation, and ocular pursuit affect how the brain integrates sensory input to produce motor output. Water learning activities should include perceptual-motor components. Rarely will a water learning session have only one goal. Each session, rather, should have a cognitive goal, a perceptual-motor goal, a social goal, a fitness or motor skill goal, and a psychological, success-oriented goal. Achievement of multiple goals results in integration of knowledge and skills.

Success Orientation

Water learning should always be fun, and what can be more fun than success? Give praise frequently. Keep the enthusiasm level high. If tasks become difficult, move to an easier task, plan a different progression, and return later to more difficult challenges. Take frequent breaks for familiar, well-liked activities and tasks. Water learning activities will be as fun and successful as adult caregivers make them. Think positively and expect to have an enjoyable experience. Success will then be the only possible result.

Universality

Water learning can be conducted anywhere by any adult caregiver. Water learning activities are easy to implement. Parents and grandparents, as well as therapists, teachers, and other caregivers can be facilitators. Each can use water learning activities to engage children in positive aquatic pursuits, creating a pleasant environment for a pool or beach experience and facilitating overall growth and development. Any adult can become a water learning facilitator.

Share water learning experiences with other caregivers. Parents, teachers, therapists, recreation personnel, and child-care staff working together can be of much greater benefit to a child than any person working alone. This is particularly important when facilitating water learning for a child with disabilities. Sharing information, particularly information on new and different activities and information on a child's accomplishments, is critical to the total team effort.

Sharing may be done through notes after an activity has been completed or during face-to-face visits between caregivers. It is important to keep notes about progress on a child or make comments regarding implementation of the activity with your class or therapy group.

Many activities are appropriate for multiple educational and therapeutic formats. Water learning in school can be continued in the bath at home. Wet fun from a recreation setting can be replicated in therapy. Therapeutic water activities can be continued in a school sink or home tub. Water is everywhere. Use it well.

Share safety procedures also. Be sure all facilitators learn the safety precautions you use during water learning. Don't count on the child remembering. Put procedures in printed form, and give copies to everyone involved. Demonstrate safety in all activity sessions. Anyone coming to observe or assist should be able to see your safety consciousness in action.

Water Learning and Swim Instruction

Most parents and children associate going to the pool, lake, or beach with learning to swim. Water learning can make a great contribution to a child's learning to swim. Learning to swim starts with an orientation to activities in water. What better way to become acquainted with activities in water than to participate in familiar activities, but in a different environment?

Water learning activities are great for water orientation, and most do not require submersion. Rather, with the problem-solving approach, the child decides whether or not to submerge. For example, submerging and grasping an object with the hand may accomplish an activity that has a goal of retrieving an object from the pool bottom. However, a child may also use his or her feet to either pick up the object or move the object to more shallow water where submersion is not necessary. As a child becomes more comfortable in water and as he or she sees other children submerge, that child may be more attracted to trying the more difficult skill. Providing helpful hints, such as "If you want to go underwater, be sure to hold your breath (or close your mouth or blow bubbles)," will make the more adventurous response easier.

For children who already have some swim skill, water learning activities can be used for warming up or tapering off a swim lesson. Challenging, as well as fun, water learning is different from swim lessons. A child having difficulty learning to swim will now have an additional and different opportunity for success.

Some children experience difficulty learning to swim because their physical fitness level is low. Water learning activities are a fun way to improve strength, endurance, and cardiorespiratory fitness. Swim skill is not required. Fitness develops as a child participates, focused on the learning task rather than striving to accomplish skills his or her body is not ready to undertake.

Where more difficult swim skills are involved, during deep-water performance, for example, focusing on an academic task rather than on skill difficulty can result in better skill performance. This is particularly true for treading water and other endurance drills. Treading water while playing a round of Uno is much more fun than just treading for time. Focus shifts to the game, and children are less conscious of the time passing in strenuous physical activity.

chapter 2

Implementing Water Learning

Water learning activities can be fantastic experiences, fun and educational for the child and enjoyable for the facilitator. However, they also can turn out to be disastrous messes, unpleasant and unsafe for the youngster and horrible for the facilitator. The secret of success is in planning and organizing ahead of time. This is not an anything goes, let's get wet time. It is structured and facilitator directed. When contemplating a water learning session, consider the physical setting and preparation for activities. Here's how.

Creating a Water Learning Environment Without a Swimming Pool

Water learning can take place at home in the bathroom or yard. Water learning can also take place in a classroom or therapy area. Water learning activities staged in the home, school, or therapy setting can be more comfortable for the child than activities in a pool setting. A small, familiar setting helps relieve anxiety. Facilitators can determine parameters, such as temperature and noise levels. Facilitators can schedule and plan water learning activities at the convenience of participants. Therefore, even if there is no access to a swimming pool, a facilitator has many options for creating a water learning environment.

Physical Setting

The physical setting for water learning activities should be an area that you don't mind getting wet. Children will drip, splash, slosh, spill, dribble, sprinkle, and otherwise get water all over the place—that is the object.

Although many activities emphasize motor control (e.g., pouring into a small container), these are learning activities. Some children will not be proficient at the outset, so learning should be fun. Fun doesn't include fussing about water getting in places it is not desired or constant reminders to keep dry items dry.

Floor surfaces should accommodate large amounts of water; a floor with a drain may be hard to come by. If using a classroom or room in a home, place a large, waterproof (not just absorbent) covering over the entire area. A small inflatable pool also works, although disposing of the water at the end of the activity might be difficult. Such a pool is probably better suited to outdoor water learning. A sponge mop can be used to mop a covering at the conclusion of the activity.

A sink, a water table, or tubs of water on a table are suitable for many activities. However, cover the floor underneath with waterproof material to avoid damaging wood or carpeted floors. Tile or cement floors could prove to be slippery when wet, making additional nonskid mats necessary.

The outdoors is an excellent setting for water play when weather cooperates. A clean, flat surface is best. Grass adds an extra textural dimension. Remember that dirt can rapidly turn to mud with the addition of water. Sand adds an extra element to creativity because water turns sand into a great building material. Working outdoors can combine water learning activities with purposeful cleanup as you and the child wash off sand, dirt, or grass after the learning event.

Air Temperature

Air should be warm enough that participants do not get chilled as they get wet. If inside, the room thermostat may need to be turned up a bit and doors and windows closed to prevent drafts. A sunny, warm day is more conducive to outdoor water learning than a cloudy, cool one. However, be sure to apply waterproof sunscreen (the higher the SPF number, the greater the protection from ultraviolet rays) to prevent sunburn. A space protected from wind is warmer than one out in the open.

A locker room or laundry room with a tile floor and several floor drains is an ideal setting for water learning. Some floors even have radiant heating under the surface. Again, check the thermostat and remove the potential for drafts.

A bathtub is a great water learning location. It is easy to clean and available to most families. As a safety precaution for activities that take place in a tub or sink, leave the drain open.

Furniture

Furniture and other objects not related to water play should be moved well out of the way. This gives the child room to be active without damaging things that aren't supposed to get wet. All furniture needed for the activity, such as chairs, bolsters, or other body-support items, should be made of waterproof materials.

Equipment

The equipment you use should be appropriate for the activity. You should be able to use all equipment in and around water without harming either the object or the child. Objects should have smooth, rather than sharp, edges. Use plastic items instead of glass. If painted, paint should be lead free. Assemble a set of items just for water learning rather than allowing children to bring familiar items to the water setting. It can be devastating to a child if a beloved toy becomes damaged during water learning. After the activity, be sure to empty and dry equipment before putting it away. Moldy equipment poses a health hazard.

Water

Set up all the buckets and tubs of water before the activity begins. It is difficult to supervise children adequately and haul water at the same time. Try to set up the activity close to the water source. If you must carry water a great distance, be careful of drips and spills in areas such as hallways where it would be not only messy but also pose a safety hazard by making floors slippery.

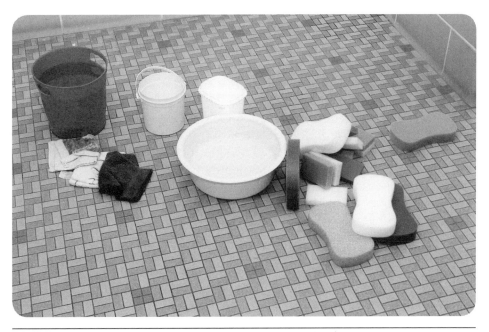

Set up the buckets and water before the activity begins.

The water you use should be clean and at a neutral temperature. Use fresh tap water to fill buckets, tubs, or other containers. Change the water if it becomes dirty. If an activity requires children to put their face into water, each child should have a personal container of water. Water at a neutral temperature is more fun to play with than cold water. Fill buckets with slightly warm (not hot, which can burn) tap water. Remember, it will cool as the children use it.

Creating a Water Learning Environment in a Swimming Pool

A swimming pool appropriate for water learning might be a backyard pool or a community swim facility. Water learning activities staged in a swimming pool allow large-muscle activity. A pool becomes a place to run and jump. A pool setting also provides more opportunities for submersion, thus paving the way for development of swim skills. Although pool size and depth may determine some activity selection, general pool characteristics are the same, no matter what the pool configuration. Use whatever pool is available.

Physical Setting

Characteristics of a pool appropriate for water learning should include clear, clean, chemically balanced water. The bottom of the pool should be conducive to physical activity by providing a nonslip surface that is not abrasive to the bottoms of feet. If the pool bottom is slippery or rough, children and facilitators can wear aquatic shoes. These shoes should not be worn outside the water environment where they could pick up dirt, sand, or grass.

Water should be waist to chest high for the children participating in the water learning program. If the pool depth is graduated, use a lifeline to separate deep water from water at the children's shoulder level. Note that this may be in addition to the lifeline at the break point separating deep water from shallow water. A lifeline placed in water above the heads of children is useless for guarding their safety.

If you will use only part of the pool for water learning, clearly mark the boundaries. Younger children may need additional lifelines. Older children, capable of monitoring where they are, may be able to note boundaries marked by cones on the deck or by backstroke flags overhead. No matter what the marking is, monitor the location of every child with ongoing surveillance to be sure none strays into water deeper than shoulder level.

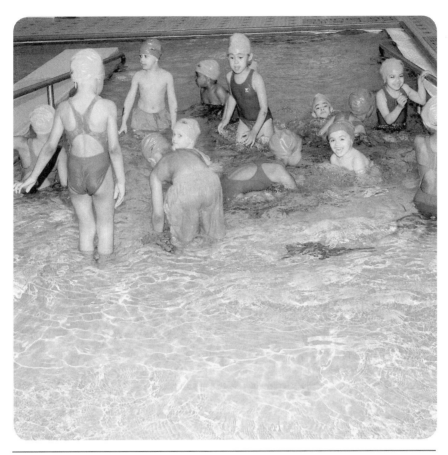

A zero-depth pool ramp allows children to choose the level of submersion they are most comfortable with.

A zero-depth pool ramp or poolside "beach" provides an additional advantage for water learning. Zero depth means water gradually increases from no depth at deck level to a depth of two to three feet (60 to 90 centimeters), thus allowing children to select the level of submersion they are most comfortable with. Zero depth also allows for kneeling, sitting, and lying on the pool bottom, positions that might not be possible in a standard pool.

Walk-in steps also provide an advantageous water learning environment. Some children might not be comfortable with total-body submersion or standing in chest-deep water. These children may sit on steps (a position that provides a firmer balance) and enter greater depth as their comfort level increases.

Air and Water Temperature

Comfort is a prime consideration. Community facilities seldom offer opportunities to adjust air and water temperature. In a community facility it is up to the facilitator to structure the water learning session to keep the child comfortable. To do this, he or she can follow these guidelines:

- Encourage the child to participate in water that is between waist and shoulder depth. Keeping more of the body underwater results in less body surface exposed to air and subject to the cooling effect of evaporation.
- Limit the time spent out of the pool. Staying in the water will keep the child warmer.
- Plan activities to keep the child moving. The more active the child, the warmer the child will be because of the increased circulation that movement provides.
- If using more sedentary activities, alternate them with highly active activities to rewarm the child.
- Select an area of the pool free from drafts if possible. Areas directly in front of doors can be drafty.

If it is possible to adjust air or water temperature, set the pool temperature at 82 to 84 degrees Fahrenheit (27.8 to 28.9 degrees Celsius). This is comfortable without being so hot that an active child will become overheated or debilitated. Air temperature should be 6 to 8 degrees Fahrenheit (3.3 to 4.4 degrees Celsius) warmer than the water temperature. Air with a relative humidity of approximately 60 percent will feel warmer than drier air. And, again, lack of drafts will keep the environment more comfortable.

Equipment

Any object can be used for water learning, provided it is child friendly and pool proof. Child friendly means it has no sharp edges, no small detachable parts, and a surface that is safe for a child to handle. Pool proof means that it is too large to pass into the pool's drain and filter systems. Pool proof also means that the pool chemicals will not destroy the object, change its color, peel surface coatings, or otherwise damage the object. A wide variety of child-friendly and pool-proof items are available, including waterproof games such as Uno, plastic toys, and foam pool equipment.

This book also describes activities that use pictures, flash cards, card games, books, and other paper objects. Although the game Uno comes in a waterproof version, most paper items do not. You can make pool versions of paper objects by laminating them. Laminating film is readily available. Use it to laminate math flash cards, a popular card game, or a picture book, and take that traditionally land-based learning activity into the pool.

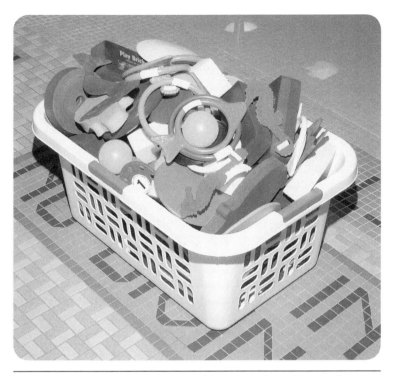

A variety of objects can be used for water learning, as long as they are child friendly and pool proof.

Creating a Water Learning Environment at a Lake or River

Many children spend time at beaches. Whether it is at a lake or ocean cottage or a campsite on a river, an open-water beach can be a great water learning setting. An appropriate setting is one with a clean beach area and clean water. Nature controls the air and water temperature. However, water learning facilitators should be sensitive to the children's comfort and take many of the same steps to assure it as they would in a pool.

Of particular importance in an open-water setting is the need to examine the site for anything hazardous to the child and remove it. This might include beach litter and animal waste as well as litter in the water, including submerged objects. Children should be able to move freely in the open-water environment without danger from environmental hazards. Be sure activity boundaries are clearly marked. Use a lifeline or enclosed pier structure to designate where a child may play safely. Teach children to refrain from chasing toys that have floated or been blown out of the area.

Preparing Participants for Water Learning

Children should wear clothing suitable for the activity. Facilitators should follow these guidelines:

- Minimal clothing is desired. Underpants only or a swimsuit is ideal. If children wear more clothing, they should have a spare set, including underwear, socks, and shoes, on hand.
- The child's clothing should be able to get wet without being damaged (e.g., tennis shoes or river sandals rather than dress shoes).
- If children wear clothing that covers their arms and legs, some total-body activities will be inappropriate.
- Each child should have his or her own towel for drying off afterward.
- After water learning activities, children should change out of wet clothing into dry items. Wearing wet clothing for a prolonged period chills the entire body.

Facilitators also need to prepare for the activity by following these guidelines:

- The child is not the only one who will get wet. Therefore, wear appropriate clothing and be ready to get as wet—or wetter—than the child.
- Be psychologically prepared to get wet. Children won't enjoy the activity if you don't. Be prepared to keep smiling, even while sitting in a puddle! Children learn by imitating behaviors. Therefore, model appropriate behavior for water activities as you interact with the child and the water. This includes enthusiasm for the activity and comfort with water.
- Plan specific activities ahead of time. Although children can and should experiment on their own, you still need to create the setting, set the ground rules, and present activity problems for the child to solve.
- Ready equipment and water ahead of time. A good facilitator is a prepared facilitator.

chapter 3

Considering Health and Safety

Because water learning can be implemented anywhere, anyone who might implement water learning activities should know how to establish and maintain a safe environment. Although water learning activities can be a great deal of fun, they can also be hazardous. Children can drown during water learning. Children can also catch diseases. Does this mean you shouldn't attempt water learning? No, of course not. However, it does mean adult facilitators must be vigilant.

Drowning Prevention

Children, particularly very young children, can drown in incredibly small amounts of water. A bucket, tub, or other container of water can be a water trap for a child who falls in headfirst. Children with disabilities in particular often cannot extricate themselves from hazards. They also sometimes cannot call out for help. Drowning can happen without a sound and in seconds. Therefore facilitators should follow these guidelines:

- Supervise all children at all times. Never leave a child unsupervised during water learning activities. This means the adult facilitator must be able to see the child at all times. If it is necessary to leave the water learning environment, another adult caregiver should take over visual supervision. If another adult is not present, take the child with you.

- When choosing a community pool setting, select a pool with a lifeguard on duty. Although not every state requires a lifeguard and some very small pools fall outside of state bathing code requirements, a pool with a certified lifeguard provides a much safer environment than an unsupervised pool does.

- If in a home or therapy pool setting, be aware that equipment in the water can obscure your view of a child underwater. Be sure to keep the child in view at all times.

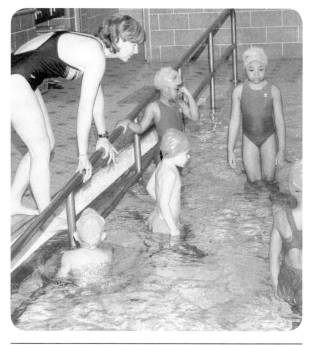

Constant supervision is a must during water learning activities.

- Be sure all equipment is in place before the child enters the environment. This includes pool safety and rescue equipment as well as water learning equipment.

- Be sure to dump all water when you have finished the activity.

- Have a phone or some other means of calling for help readily available. Keep emergency contact information with the phone.

- You should be certified in infant and child cardiopulmonary resuscitation and should renew that certification every year.

- Teach every child water safety rules. Help the child learn them through reminders and active enforcement during each water learning session. Those rules should include, but are not limited to, the following:

  An adult must be present when you are playing in or around water.

  Do not start to play with the water learning equipment until an adult tells you to begin.

  Move slowly and carefully when moving on a wet surface.

- In a nonpool venue, remember that sitting or kneeling is a safer position for activity than standing is.

Contagion

Tap and swimming pool water, in and of themselves, do not make people sick. However, what people put in water can make it infectious. Equipment used for water learning is not dangerous. However, equipment can become contaminated during use. Germs cannot be seen, and people can spread them without knowing it. Unwell people can seem healthy and yet be carrying disease germs. It is always safe to view each person involved in water learning as contagious. Therefore, in the nonpool environment, each child should have his or her own water supply and toys if the following occurs:

- The activity involves putting the face in the water.
- The child has an open wound on his or her body.
- Any of the equipment is to be put into the mouth.
- The child drools or has a drippy nose.
- The child has a contagious condition.

In a pool environment, a child should not participate if any of the following occur:

- The child has an open wound on his or her body.
- The child has a contagious condition.
- The child has diarrhea.

Furthermore, a child should not share pool equipment if any of the following occur:

- Any of the equipment is to be put into the mouth.
- The child drools or has a drippy nose.

For most water learning activities, children can share equipment and water. Sharing is part of learning to play and work with other people. When equipment or water will be shared, considering the following guidelines will help keep everyone healthy:

- Do not share equipment if it will be put into the mouth.
- Children who drool or have drippy noses should not share equipment.

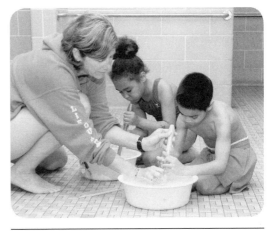

For health reasons, ensure that children do not share equipment that is put into the mouth.

After completing activities involving shared equipment, clean all equipment with soap and water and dry it. In addition, equipment that has been put into the mouth and equipment that has come in contact with bodily fluids, including blood, urine, feces, saliva, nasal discharge, and vomit, should be cleaned with a solution of half a cup of liquid chlorine bleach to one gallon (4.5 liters) of fresh water (1 part bleach to 10 parts water) (American Red Cross 2006) using the following procedure:

1. Wear gloves while handling used equipment.
2. Soak the equipment in the water and bleach solution for a minimum of 10 minutes.
3. Wash the equipment in soap and water.
4. Rinse the equipment in clear water.
5. Dry the equipment.
6. Store equipment in a clean and dry area.

Injury Prevention

Many water learning activities use everyday household items. This is one of the wonderful aspects of water learning outside of the pool environment—no special equipment is needed. However, keep in mind that household items are not intended to be used as toys by small children. Therefore, facilitators must exercise judgment when selecting equipment. Before each water learning session, check all equipment. Do not use equipment with sharp edges, corners, or pieces. Be sure all parts of the equipment are securely attached (e.g., pot handles are on pots, bucket handles are on buckets). Make sure the size of the objects is appropriate for the child's age and behavior. Do not use an object that the child could put in his or her mouth and swallow or choke on. If the object is painted, be sure the paint is not peeling and is lead free.

In a pool environment, the equipment must be safe for the child and appropriate for the setting. Equipment shown on the following page is designed specifically for use in swimming pools, or made of material safe for pool use.

Do not use equipment that will disintegrate in the pool. Promptly remove equipment that shows signs of disintegration. For example, immediately remove a foam noodle that starts to flake off foam, and find it a new home in the trash. Do not use equipment that bleeds dye into the water. Do not use an object with sharp edges; this equipment could not only injure a child but also puncture a pool lining. All equipment should be large enough to not pass into a drain.

Emergency action planning is an important part of injury prevention. Everyone needs an emergency action plan (EAP), a detailed description

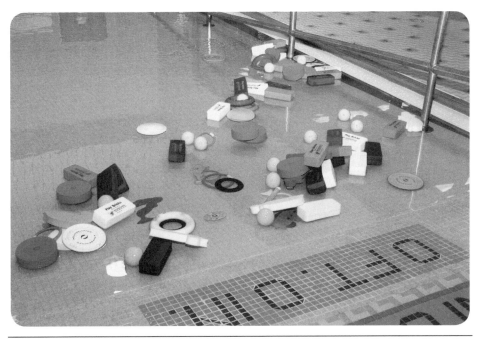

Having a wide variety of equipment will enable many different water learning activities.

of what should be done in the case of a life-threatening emergency or serious illness. You should plan and document all procedures, beginning from the point of recognition of the situation and ending with what to do after emergency medical services (EMS) personnel leave the scene.

In a pool environment, the facility should already have an EAP. This document is part of normal pool operations. The EAP details the responsibilities of staff during an emergency. In a home, school, or therapy water learning setting, having an EAP is the responsibility of the parent, teacher, or therapist, as part of ensuring participant safety.

The EAP is activated by the person who recognizes the emergency. The answers to these questions should be documented in the plan:

- Who calls EMS (from which phone, giving what directions)?
- Who provides emergency care to the victim?
- Who provides supervision and care to the rest of the children?
- Who goes to meet EMS personnel?
- Who notifies parents (if necessary)?
- Who documents the situation?
- Who is responsible for making changes so that this emergency does not occur again (if appropriate)?

A home EAP won't be quite the same as one for a school, therapy, or recreation setting. But any plan will contain the major components. Print out the plan, give it to all facilitators, and practice it in drill form (just like a fire drill). Leave a printed copy next to the phone you will use to call EMS along with the other information that someone calling EMS will need (e.g., address, phone number, entrance to use).

Child safety is important. One emergency is enough to handle. Failure to take additional precautions during an emergency could result in additional harm and possible loss of life. Be prepared. Have, know, and practice your EAP.

Swimming Pool Safety

Safe participation is the first goal of any water learning program. Water learning activities must be staged safely. A pool environment can be a wonderful venue for child growth and development. That same environment can turn deadly in mere seconds. Although water learning pool activities can take place in a small therapy pool, a backyard pool, a bathtub, a wading pool, or a Hubbard tank, for purposes of discussing safety, we will assume you are using a standard community pool. If the environment is smaller than this, you may make modifications as long as you do not compromise the basic premise of the safety precaution.

- Use a facility that is in compliance with all local municipality health and safety codes.
- Follow all of the facility's health and safety rules, including suit, cap, and shower requirements.
- Make sure a lifeguard with current certification at the national level is on duty at all times. Participant surveillance and emergency response should be the lifeguard's only duties.
- Prepare and set up equipment before the children enter the pool area.

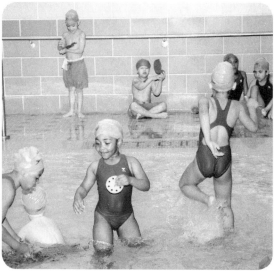

Preparing equipment takes time. Plan for setup before children arrive.

- Teach children pool rules, and actively enforce those rules with reminders, cues, behavior modeling, praise, positive reinforcement, time-outs, and exclusions as necessary.
- Teach children to enter the water only when the adult accompanying them gives permission. They should learn to wait for this direction.
- Interact with children and supervise them during the entire water learning session. Remember, water learning consists of structured activity. Children interacting with adults are safe.
- Plan age-appropriate activities. Children who are encouraged to try activities beyond their age or ability level can easily become injured or fearful.
- Consider readiness when planning activities. Do not force children into activities for which they are not physically and psychologically ready.
- Because water learning activities are designed to take place at a depth that participants can stand in (as opposed to deep water), modify activities as necessary so that children with physical disabilities always have a safe resting place at the side of the pool or on a support platform.
- Let the child choose whether to completely submerge or not. If you notice that a child is not able to control breath holding or is drinking water, caution the child to close his or her mouth, and limit submersions to no more than three per session.

Water learning is also suitable for a backyard pool, either in ground or above ground, a wading pool, or a lake or river waterfront. If you are using one of these environments, follow these guidelines:

- An adult with current certification in CPR and first aid should be with the children at all times (in lieu of a lifeguard).
- A phone should be available at the water.
- All safety precautions related to the water learning activities stated earlier apply.
- If the venue is outside, be sure appropriate precautions are taken against sunburn. (Even dark-skinned children can sunburn.)

Lake Safety

Summer brings many different types of water learning opportunities. Trips to the beach or vacation cottage often include experiences in open water—that lake, pond, or river we remember from our childhood. You can include water learning activities on the vacation agenda. Here's how:

- Plan specific activities appropriate to the vacation setting.
- Pack water learning toys and necessary equipment.
- Check the water environment to be sure it is safe. This includes clear, clean water, free of litter and natural debris. Avoid areas with strong waves and currents.
- Walk in the water where the child will be active. Check for sharp objects under the water and for submerged litter.
- Check the entire area for animal waste.
- Remember sunscreen.

A visit to grandma and grandpa can include water learning. This is a great opportunity to give relatives a chance to have significant interaction with a child and at the same time provide excellent learning activities that are fun for everyone.

part II

Water Learning
Activities

Opportunities for water learning are varied and numerous. To aid in planning and implementation, we have divided water learning activities into two groups based on the setting. Chapter 4 presents activities that take place somewhere besides a swimming pool. Chapter 5 includes water learning activities that take place in a swimming pool. Each chapter begins with a description of a typical activity session. In chapter 4, activities are arranged in alphabetical order by the name of the activity. In chapter 5 they are arranged by the type of equipment used.

The activity finder on pages v to xvi provides an index of developmental areas that are reinforced so that facilitators can locate activities specific to the learning needs of the child. It also provides an equipment index so that facilitators can locate activities that use particular types of equipment. Be sure to keep notes about each child's progress and activity implementation.

chapter 4

Water Learning Activities for the Nonpool Environment

Planning a nonpool water learning activity session begins by determining goals for 5-year-old Mario. He is working on improving hand, arm, and shoulder strength to better facilitate grasp and release, holding objects, and carrying. Mario is in kindergarten and is just starting to do easy addition problems. To help Mario improve in the selected areas, his facilitator looks at the learning reinforced section of the activity finder (pages v to xiii), and, based on Mario's needs, chooses Pour and Fill, Scoop and Fill, Pick Up Chips, and Wring Out as the activities for the day.

Because it is summer and warm outside, the activities will take place on the patio. While Mario is finishing a snack, his facilitator places on the patio several buckets of various sizes along with a large tub of water, a washcloth, a sponge, a cup, a ladle, a bowl, a clean empty milk carton, and a dozen poker chips. Mario's facilitator then changes into shorts and a T-shirt, and helps Mario put on his swimsuit. After dressing, Mario's facilitator picks up the cordless phone and both go to the patio.

For the next 30 minutes, Mario solves movement problems set by his facilitator, who asks the following:

Can you use the sponge to get water from the tub to fill the cup?

Can you use the washcloth to get water from the tub to fill the cup?

Can you use the ladle to get water from the tub to fill the cup?

Note: The progression is from an object easy to grasp (the sponge) to one more difficult to grasp and control (the ladle). Mario's facilitator encourages him during the more difficult aspects of the task and allows him to experiment with the other scooping and pouring items available.

Can you use the same scoopers to fill a bucket?

Note: Now the progression is to fill a larger container.

Can you use the cup to fill the bucket?

Can you use a small bucket to fill the larger bucket?

Note: Now Mario must lift and carry something heavy.

Can you use the same tools to empty the bucket?

Can you think of a faster way to empty the bucket?

Note: Here the progression starts with a larger amount of water and ends with a total water dump.

The session isn't over yet. Now that Mario is quite wet from the bucket dump, he and his facilitator also try Pick Up Chips. This activity requires more concentration because Mario must add and count in addition to identifying color and grasping small objects. Because Mario is a bit hyperactive, his facilitator saved this task for after the scooping and pouring, recognizing that Mario would do better if he spent some of his pent-up energy before having to concentrate.

Finally, Mario and his facilitator also try some of the activities from the previous water learning session. Sponge Off was a favorite. **Note:** Return to an easier and more fun task at the end of the session to be sure to end on a positive note.

At the end of the session, Mario's facilitator takes him to get dressed and to lie down for a nap. When Mario is inside, warm, dry, and settled, the facilitator returns to the patio to clean up after the activity. Finally, the facilitator makes notes in Mario's activity book to document progress and to aid in planning for the next session.

Big and Little

Learning Reinforced

Concepts of big and little, finger dexterity, grasp and release

Equipment

Large bucket of water, objects matched for big and little that sink (e.g., large and small poker chips, large and small blocks, large and small alphabet letters)

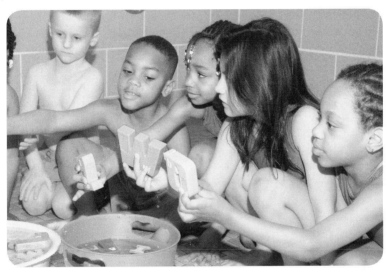

Description

Place all objects into the bucket, and ask the child if he or she can find a *big* or *little* one. It may be necessary to show the child the objects and describe them first. Praise successful selections, and reinforce the child by saying, "Yes, you have a *big* (or *little*) block." If the selection is incorrect, ask the child to hold up his or her object, and then hold the appropriately sized object next to the one the child is holding. Discuss the difference between the child's object and the object that is the correct size. Try the activity again.

Variations

Place all objects into the bucket. Select one, and show it to the child. Ask the child to tell you if you have a big one or a little one. Then ask the child if he or she can find an object that matches yours. When the child makes a selection, ask if he or she has a big or a little object. To increase difficulty, have the child try the original selection problem blindfolded. Matching objects that have cognitive meaning, such as big and little alphabet letters, adds the additional task of letter recognition. Ask the child, "Can you tell me what letter this is?" and follow with "Is it a big or little _____?"

Block Sort

Learning Reinforced

Shape discrimination, shape matching, finger dexterity and strength, grasp and release, concepts of floating and of fit

Equipment

Large bucket of water, blocks of different shapes, shape container (a container with holes of different shapes that correspond to the shape of the blocks)

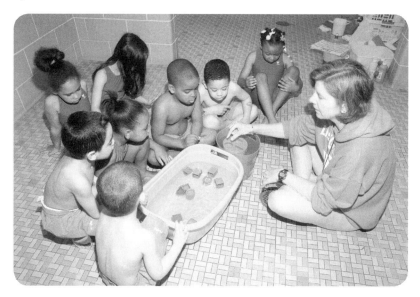

Description

Place the empty shape container in the bucket, filling and submerging the shape container. Allow the blocks to float in the bucket alongside the container. Ask the child, "Can you put the blocks into the container?" If a block is inserted correctly, praise the child, saying "Yes, that one fits!" If the child makes an incorrect selection and cannot push the block into the container, ask the child, "Does that one fit? No? Can you try a different block?" Be sure the container remains underwater so that the child has to push the shapes in. Most plastic blocks float if not forced into the container. It is important to let the child try any block he or she selects, even if you know it will not work. The child must reach the same conclusion by trying rather than being told.

Variations

Ask the child to name the shape of the block he or she selects. This activity may be more challenging if the child is blindfolded.

Blow

Learning Reinforced

Concept and motor skill of blowing and breath control

Equipment

Small bucket of water, straw, blow tube, plastic saxette or plastic recorder (You can make a blow tube by taking either a plastic tube, like one used to hold golf clubs in a bag or a piece of plastic disposable tubing from a respiratory therapy machine, and cutting it into sections two to three inches [5.1 to 7.6 centimeters] long; each section makes one blow tube.)

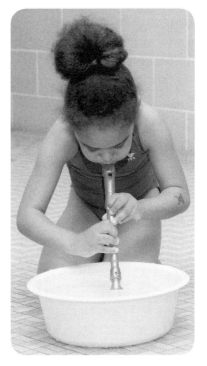

Description

Ask the child to put one end of the tube into his or her mouth and hold it there. Then put the other end into the water, and ask the child, "Can you blow bubbles?" It may be easier for some children to hold one end in the water. Encourage the child by asking, "Can you take a breath and blow out through the tube?" Use the wider tube first and then try the straw. Do not allow the child to drink the water.

Variation

Some children cannot differentiate between blowing and inhaling. Everyone who breathes without mechanical assistance is already blowing when they exhale. When you teach children how to blow, you are teaching them to differentiate between exhaling and inhaling, and then to be able to consciously exhale with force on command. To help children learn the difference, use a saxette. Have the children put the mouthpiece into their mouth. Then help them cover all of the holes with their fingers (or your fingers). Ask them to blow. When they do, they will hear a sound. Vary the pitch of the sound by uncovering different holes.

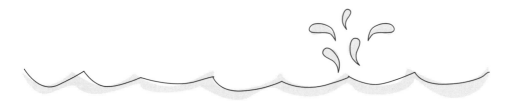

Body Painting

Learning Reinforced

Body awareness, body-part identification, color recognition, daily living activities, washing

Equipment

Small paintbrushes, watercolor paint (tempera) or finger paint in the primary colors, color cards in primary colors, small plastic containers for paint, large bucket of water, watering can or shower

Description

Put a small amount of paint into a plastic container. Use one container for each paint color. Give the child a brush and ask him or her to select a color and mark his or her foot with that color. Name different body parts and different colors. Name or ask the child to name the body part and the color as painting occurs. Show a color card as a visual cue instead of giving a verbal cue. Or show the card as you say the color name.

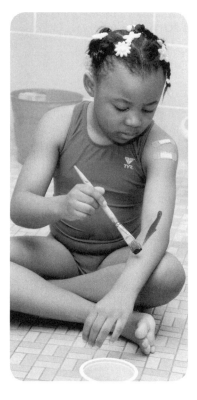

If children name a body part or color incorrectly, ask them, "Are you sure?" If children try again and answer correctly, praise their correct choice. If the new answer is incorrect, say, "Good guess; however, this is really _____." Then return to that body part or color later. Children should shower or use a watering can to wash off the paint. While sprinkling the child, ask, "Can you wash the paint off your ____ (name the body part you want the child to wash)?"

Safety Tip

In this and any other activity using paint, check ahead of time to be sure the child does not have paint allergies. Also, if the activity takes place at school, make sure all paint is washed off before the child goes home. If parents are not present for the activity, point out residual paint marks and describe the activity.

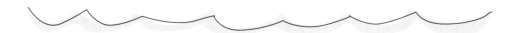

Variation

Add plastic containers for mixing paint. Start with primary colors (red, yellow, blue) and ask the child to mix colors to get green, purple, and orange. When learning the matching body parts, begin by painting one member of a body-part pair a certain color and then ask the child to paint the matching body part the same color. (Note that painting a body part means marking that part with a color. It does not mean totally covering it with paint). For children able to handle a paintbrush with ease, encourage painting body parts with flowers, stars, shapes, letters, numbers, and other easily recognizable figures.

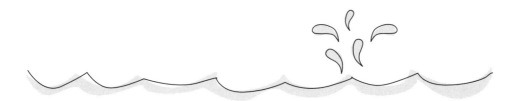

Bristle Blocks

Learning Reinforced

Finger dexterity, finger strength, grasp and release, color recognition, counting

Equipment

Bucket of water, one set of bristle blocks (blocks that stick together)

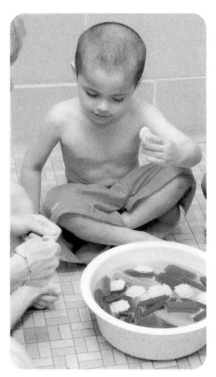

Description

Clump bristle blocks together, and drop them into the water. Ask the child, "Can you pull off one block?" Ask for blocks of different colors. Ask for a specific number of blocks.

Variations

This activity can also be done with snap beads, Peabody chips, or any other objects that can be connected and pulled apart.

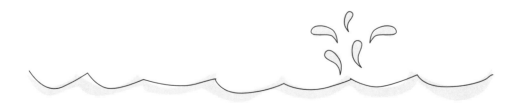

Carton Pour

Learning Reinforced

Hand and arm strength and endurance, eye–hand coordination, concepts of empty and full and of capacity

Equipment

Several clean, empty half-pint, quart, and half-gallon (0.25-, 1-, and 2-liter) milk cartons, several large buckets of water

Description

Ask the child if he or she can use a small carton to fill one of the larger cartons with water from the bucket. If the child has difficulty planning how to accomplish the task, break the problem into smaller parts by first asking the child to dip a small milk carton into the bucket and scoop up water. Then ask the child if he or she can empty the small carton into the large carton without spilling any water. Encourage the child to repeat the tasks until one of the larger cartons is filled.

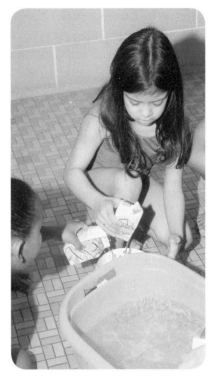

Variation

Have the child pour water from one carton to another—emptying one and filling the other. Gradually work up to pouring from larger and larger cartons. Vary the sizes so that eventually the child fills several small cartons with the contents of the largest carton. Then discuss the relationship between the size of the carton and the amount of water it will hold.

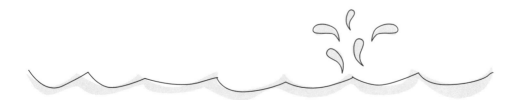

Cleanup

Learning Reinforced

Concepts of washing and cleanup, hand and arm strength and endurance, body image, daily living activities

Equipment

Brown or black tempera or finger paint (to simulate dirt), large bucket of water, one paintbrush, sponge or washcloth

Description

Paint a mark on a waterproof surface on the floor. Ask the child, "Can you use your washcloth (or sponge) to clean up this mess?" Encourage the child to dip the cloth in water, rub hard on the mark, and rinse and wring out the cloth.

> ### *Safety Tip*
>
> In this and any other activity using paint, check ahead of time to be sure the child using the paint has no paint allergies. Also, be sure all paint is removed before the child goes home (if done at school). If parents are not present for the activity, it might be wise to notify parents of any residual paint marks.

Variation

Paint marks on body parts and ask the child to clean them with a washcloth or sponge. When you mark a body part, ask the child, "What is this?" As the child cleans the body part, ask, "What part of your body are you washing?" Encourage the child to dip the cloth in water, rub hard on the mark, and rinse and wring out the cloth.

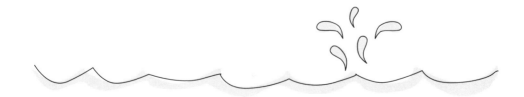

Color Bucket Sort

Learning Reinforced

Color recognition, grasp and release, color matching, sorting

Equipment

Several buckets in different colors filled with water, blocks or other objects in colors that match the buckets

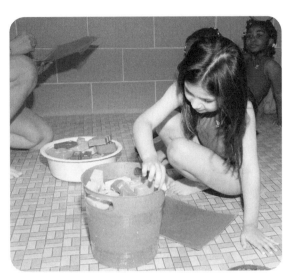

Description

Place the blocks or objects on the floor in front of the child. Ask the child to sort the objects by color into the appropriate buckets. Next, place all the objects into a single bucket of water, and ask the child to sort the objects by color into the appropriate buckets.

Variations

Add number concepts to the challenge by asking the child to sort specific numbers of specific color blocks.

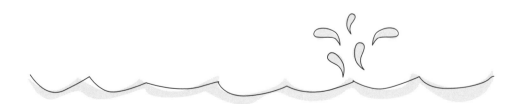

Dry Brush Body Painting

Learning Reinforced

Body awareness, body-part identification, kinesthetic awareness

Equipment

Paintbrush

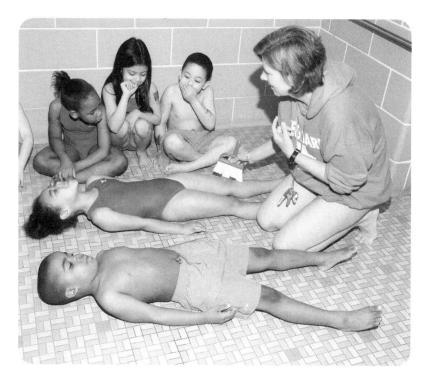

Description

Use a dry brush and paint different body parts with invisible paint. Name the part you are painting. Ask the child, "Can you wiggle the part I paint?" Ask the child to tell you the part he or she is wiggling.

Variations

Ask one child to use invisible paint to paint a body part on another child. Make a game of the activity by seeing if you (or a child) can paint a body part that the child being painted cannot name. Then teach the name of the new part, and have the children reverse roles. You can also ask the child to paint parts of your body. Try the activity with the child blindfolded for increased kinesthetic awareness.

Face Dunks

Learning Reinforced
Breath control

Equipment
Shallow tub of water

Description
Ask the child, "Can you put your chin in the water?" Ask the child to place his or her mouth in the water. Ask the child to place his or her hair in the water. Gradually work up to placing his or her entire face in the water. For sanitary reasons, each child should have his or her own tub of clean water.

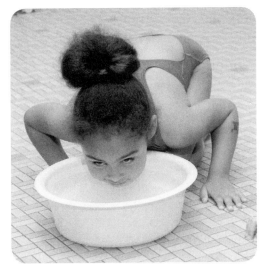

Variation
To assist children who may not feel comfortable placing parts of their face in water, ask first if they can wash the respective facial areas.

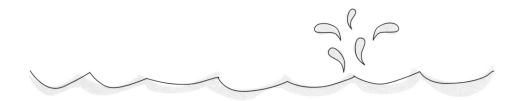

Face Dunks and Bubbles

Learning Reinforced
Breath control, blowing

Equipment
Shallow tub of water

Description
Ask the child, "Can you put your mouth near the water and blow to make bubbles?" Gradually work up to having the child put his or her whole face in the water and blow bubbles. Blowing through the mouth is easier to start. Blowing through the nose will keep

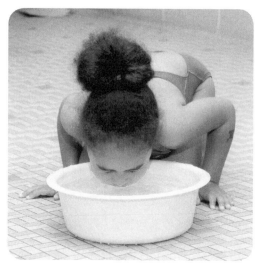

water from entering the nose and possibly being inhaled. Blowing through both the mouth and nose requires the most skill. For sanitary reasons, be sure each child has his or her own tub of clean water.

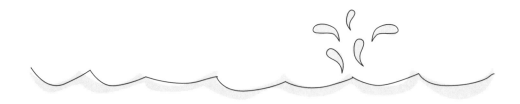

Face Dunks and Counting

Learning Reinforced

Breath control, counting, blowing

Equipment

Shallow tub of water

Description

Ask the child to do Face Dunks or Face Dunks and Bubbles. While the child keeps his or her face in the water, you count out loud to a predetermined number. Start with one or two counts and work up.

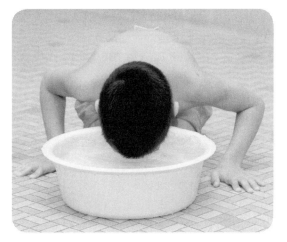

Variations

Ask the child, "Can you guess how long you can blow?" Or count silently and when the child comes up, ask, "Can you guess how long you blew bubbles?"

Safety Tip

Children should breathe normally before they hold their breath. Do not encourage them to breathe more deeply in an attempt to stay under longer. Do not encourage them to hold their breath longer than 30 seconds.

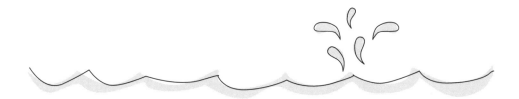

Fill the Bucket

Learning Reinforced

Hand and arm strength and endurance, finger dexterity, grasp and squeeze, empty and full

Equipment

Sponges of different sizes, large bucket of water, small empty bucket

Description

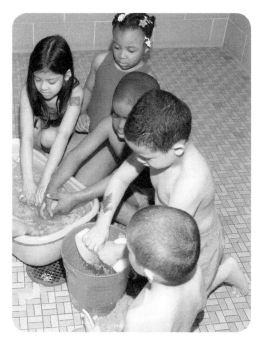

Ask the child, "Can you use your sponge to take water from the large bucket and fill the small bucket?" The child should be able to soak the sponge in water, hold the sponge over the small bucket, and squeeze it or wring it out. Continue this process until the small bucket is full of water. If the challenge is too difficult, divide the task into smaller parts: "Can you soak your sponge? Good job. Now can you hold your sponge over the empty bucket? Yes, that's the place. Now, can you squeeze your sponge and let the water run into the empty bucket? Can you do it again to fill the bucket?" Start with small sponges and gradually work up to large sponges. When the bucket is full, reverse the process and soak the sponge in the full bucket and wring it out over a drain, continuing until the bucket is empty again.

Variations

Use each hand singly and both hands together. Older children can fill and empty the bucket against a time limit. Each session they should try to better their previous times. This increases the workload on hands and forearms, thus improving strength and endurance. Periodically ask the child to lift the bucket with one or both hands and estimate how full it is (half, almost, not very). This increases their comprehension of the concepts of empty and full.

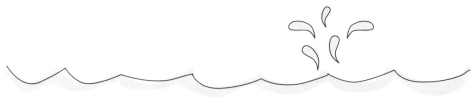

Find the Food

Learning Reinforced

Object identification, matching, identifying food and cooking items

Equipment

Large bucket of water, toy tea set, toy cooking set, plastic toy food (sometimes included in tea sets and cooking sets; refrigerator magnets sold in cooking stores also work)

Description

Place food, toy tea set, and cooking set in the water. Ask the child to find all the food or all the pots and pans. After the child becomes familiar with the items, ask for them by specific names. For example, "Can you find the peas?" or "Can you find something to go with this cup?"

Variations

Have pictures of the food or cooking set, and ask the child if he or she can find the item that matches the picture. For another variation, ask the child to find the item you describe, for example, "Can you find what we drink out of?" Older children can learn more complicated matches. For example, show the child a cooking pot, and ask if he or she can find something that could be cooked in that pot.

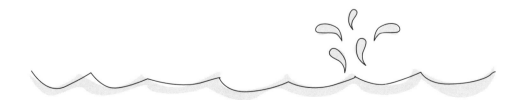

Flat and Round

Learning Reinforced
Finger dexterity, concepts of flat and round

Equipment
Large bucket of water, poker chips, balls

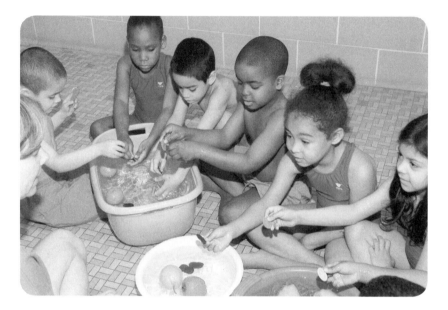

Description
Put objects into the bucket, and ask the child if he or she can find a flat or round object. It may be necessary to show the child the items and label them before placing them in the bucket. Having one of each type of item outside the bucket for a match may also be helpful.

Variations
Add the concept of color by asking, "Can you pick up something blue and flat? Can you find something round and red?" Try this activity blindfolded.

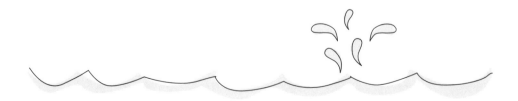

Full and Empty

Learning Reinforced

Concepts of empty and full, hand and arm strength and endurance, concept of capacity

Equipment

A variety of containers of different sizes, large bucket of water, cup, scoop or ladle

Description

Ask the child if he or she can fill one of the containers by using a cup to transfer water from the bucket to the container.

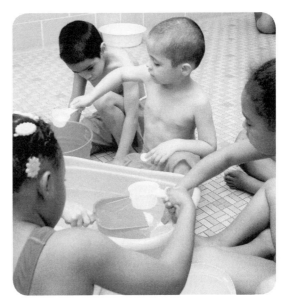

Variations

Vary the sizes of the containers the children will fill and the implements they will use. Reverse the process and ask the children to empty the containers back into the tub. For highly skilled children, ask them to fill the container half full, one-quarter full, and one-third full. Discuss which containers hold more water than others. Experiment with containers of irregular shapes, and try to guess which container will hold more or how many scoops it will take to fill the container.

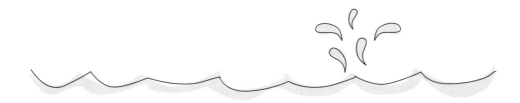

Hair Wash

Learning Reinforced

Hair washing, daily living activities

Equipment

Large bucket of water, sponges, cups, watering can or other items to pour water over the head

Description

Ask the child, "Can you get ready to wash your hair?" Make believe that you are washing the hair by pouring water over the child's head. Start with just a sprinkle and work up to larger amounts of water. Initially, aim low on the side or back of the head. Gradually, as the child's comfort increases, move higher on the head and forward so that water actually runs down the face. Ask the child, "Can you help me get you wet all over?" Offer the child sponges, a cup, or other items for pouring so he or she can help. If the child enjoys this, actually soap up and then rinse.

Safety Tips

- If you will use soap, check with the home caregivers first to determine if there are allergies or a shampoo preference. Be sure hair is dry before going outside, especially in cold weather. If you use soap, be sure all of it is rinsed out before drying the hair.

- Take special precautions with a child who has ear tubes. He or she should wear earplugs during this activity so that no water enters the ear canals.

Variations

To further ease any reticence on the part of the child, allow the child to perform the same tasks as you. Have fun washing each other's hair!

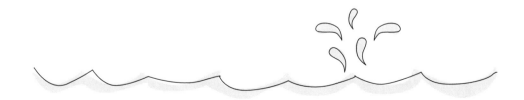

Hammering

Learning Reinforced

Grasp and squeeze, hand and arm strength and endurance, eye–hand coordination, hammering

Equipment

Plastic workbench or cobbler's bench with pegs and hammer, shallow tub of water

Description

Place the bench in a tub of water so that the holes are one-half to one inch (1.3 to 2.4 centimeters) below the water surface. Ask the child, "Can you use the hammer to pound the pegs through the holes, just like when you use the bench out of the water?" Encourage the child to continue hammering even though it causes splashing as the hammer hits the water.

Variations

Ask the child to hammer pegs of a specific color into specific holes. Ask the child to hammer a specific number of pegs.

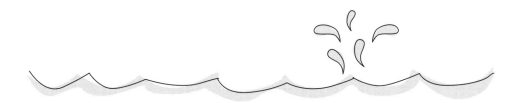

Hand and Foot Prints

Learning Reinforced
Body-part identification

Equipment
Construction paper, shallow tub of water

Description
Ask the child, "Can you make a handprint (or footprint)?" To further facilitate this task, ask the child to dip a hand or foot in the water. Then cue him or her to shake off excess water over the water bucket and not over the paper. Finally, ask "Now, can you press your hand onto the paper and make a print?" Remember to keep the paper in a dry place so that only the body part makes a wet print.

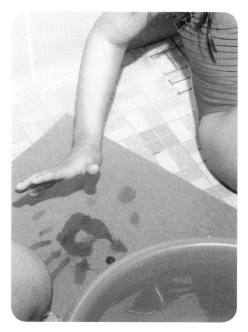

Variations
Label and identify left and right. Make prints of other dunkable body parts, such as an elbow, chin, or toe.

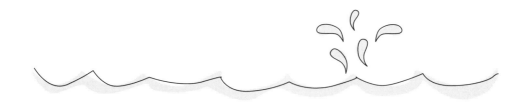

Ice Fishing

Learning Reinforced

Concept of temperature, grasp and release, finger dexterity

Equipment

One or two trays of ice cubes, objects that sink, large bucket of water

Description

Place objects in the tub, then add the ice cubes. Ask the child, "Can you reach through the ice cubes and find _____ (name an object)?" As the child reaches into the water, he or she might be surprised by the cold temperature. Reinforce the child's observations by asking "How does that feel?" and to the child's response add "Yes, that is really different. That's cold."

Variations

You can add ice to almost any water learning activity involving object retrieval. Changing the character of the water not only increases the difficulty but also adds stimulation to the body surfaces immersed. Do not add ice to activities in which the children place their face in water or you pour water over them.

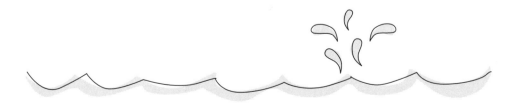

Paint Mix

Learning Reinforced

Color recognition, finger dexterity, grasp and release, cleanup, daily living activities

Equipment

Large bucket of water; several small paper cups or shallow plastic dishes; small paintbrushes; watercolor paint in red, yellow, and blue

Description

Ask the child, "Can you mix paint to make the color green?" Help the child use the small cups for mixing different paint colors. Be sure to use clean water between

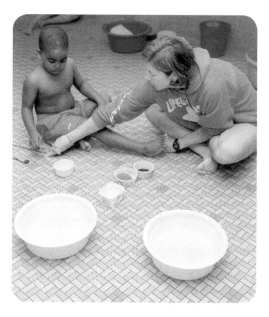

colors and on brushes to avoid ending up with brown paint. Follow this activity with Cleanup (see page 46).

Variations

Use parts of the body as pallets for mixing paint. Place a small dab of yellow paint on the top of a foot, for example. Then place a dab of blue over the dab of yellow, and mix with a brush to see what color the foot becomes.

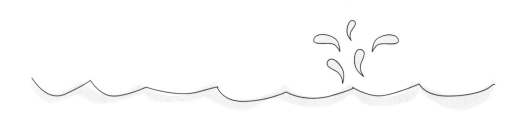

Pick Up Chips

Learning Reinforced

Finger dexterity, grasp and release, color recognition, counting, math concepts

Equipment

Bucket of water, poker chips of various colors

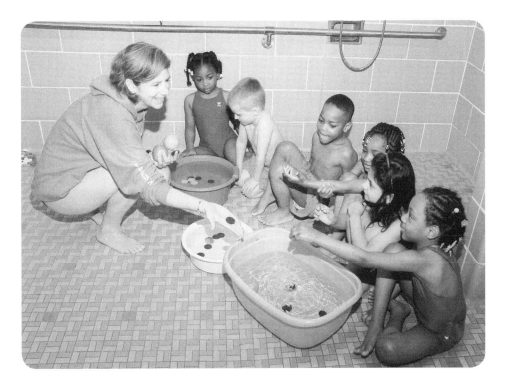

Description

Scatter chips on the bottom of a bucket of water. Ask the child, "Can you pick up a chip?" You can designate a color or a number of chips to pick up.

Variations

To make the task more difficult, give two-part directions: "Can you pick up two white chips and one blue chip?" For an even more difficult challenge, turn the pickup into a math problem: "Can you pick up the total of four chips and two chips?" The child can also do this activity blindfolded for additional challenge.

Picture Identification

Learning Reinforced

Object identification, visual discrimination, memory, breath control

Equipment

Shallow tub of water, laminated pictures of objects or animals

Description

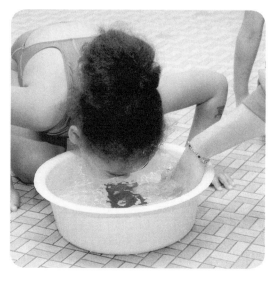

Place a picture on the bottom of the tub of water and gently ruffle the water so that the child cannot see the picture. Ask the child, "Can you put your face in the tub, take a look, come back up, and tell what you see?" Begin with simple pictures of single items, gradually increasing the detail of the picture as the child's skill underwater improves.

Variation

When the child tells you what he or she sees, ask additional questions about picture details. If the child remembers the details, praise his or her good memory. If the child does not remember, ask, "Can you take another look?"

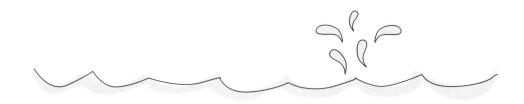

Pour and Fill

Learning Reinforced

Hand and arm strength and endurance, eye–hand coordination, concepts of empty and full

Equipment

A variety of objects useful for pouring, several containers of different sizes with openings of different sizes, a large bucket of water

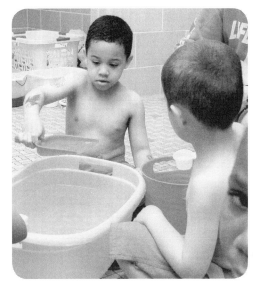

Description

Ask the child, "Can you fill the empty _____?" To further assist a child who may have difficulty planning the entire task, break the task into smaller parts by asking "Can you fill _____ (name a pouring object) from the large bucket of water? Good, now can you pour it to fill one of the other containers?" Start with large-mouthed containers first, gradually working toward containers with small openings. If the child pours successfully, praise the child for careful pouring. If pouring is messy, do not criticize. Rather, encourage more careful pouring by asking, "Can you pour without spilling quite so much?"

Variations

Ask more advanced children to estimate how many times they will have to fill and pour from one container to fill another. Increase the challenge by asking the child to pour without spilling water. Time the filling effort to add a speed component to the task.

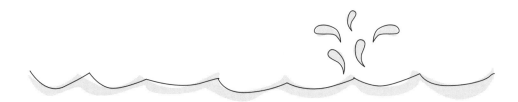

Round and Square

Learning Reinforced
Finger dexterity, concepts of round and square

Equipment
Small blocks and balls that sink, a bucket of water

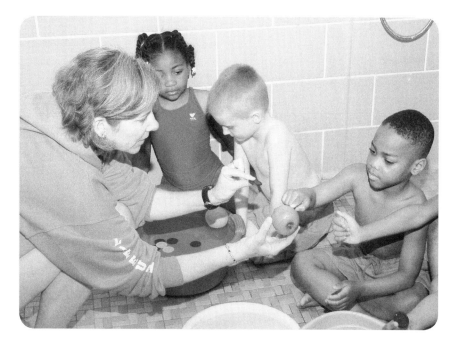

Description
Place objects into the bucket. Ask the child, "Can you pick up a round (or square) object?" It may be necessary to show items to the child and explain them first.

Variations
To increase difficulty, have the child work blindfolded. If the child can count, ask for a specific number of square objects and a specific number of round objects. Mix the number of square and round objects in one challenge, "Can you pick up two round and three square objects?"

Soap Up

Learning Reinforced

Body-part identification, washing, daily living activities

Equipment

Several buckets of water, soap (check for allergies and soap preferences), watering cans, washcloth

Description

Ask the child to name and then soap individual body parts. Begin by asking, "Can you tell me what this _____ (point to the child's knee) is?" If the child responds "my knee," reply, "Can you soap your knee?" If the child gives an incorrect response, say "That isn't your foot. That is your knee." Avoid the word *no.* It does not supply information. Give information to aid future decision making. After the body parts are soaped, use the watering can and washcloth to wash off the soap. You can also rinse the whole body with a hose and shower attachment if the activity is outside or in a locker room.

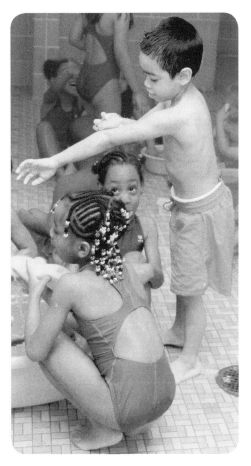

Variation

Use small containers to hold soap lather mixed with watercolors. Apply different colors to different body parts.

Scoop and Fill

Learning Reinforced

Eye–hand coordination, hand and arm strength and endurance, concept of empty and full

Equipment

Large bucket of water, small empty bucket, small scoops or shovels of different sizes

Description

Ask the child, "Can you fill the small bucket with water by scooping water out of the large bucket and into the small one?"

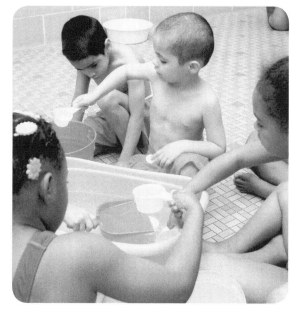

Variations

Gradually increase the distance between the buckets so that the child must carry the scoop or hold it longer. Encourage the child not to spill. As the smaller bucket fills with water, ask the child, "How full is the small bucket now?" Encourage answers that quantify, such as "The small bucket is half full," or "The small bucket is almost all full." Praise successful results.

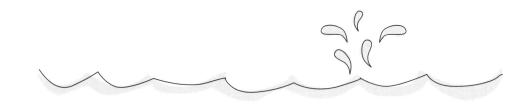

Shape Cleanup

Learning Reinforced

Hand and arm strength and endurance, concept of cleanup, shape and letter recognition, spelling, daily living activities

Equipment

Foam or plastic geometric shapes or letters that have gotten dirty through use (or mark them with brown finger paint to simulate dirt), mild soap, bucket of wash water, bucket of rinse water

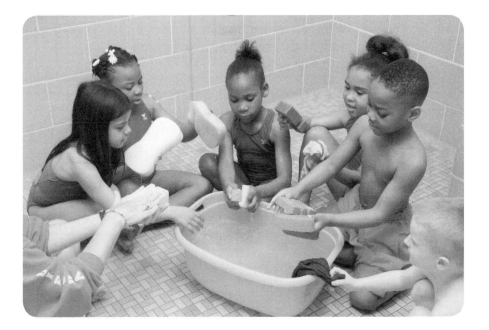

Description

Ask the child, "Can you clean these shapes?" Be sure the child squeezes the foam shapes to get the soapy water into them to clean them and also squeezes them to rinse them. It may be necessary to explain the difference between wash and rinse.

Variations

Name the shape as the child washes it. If the shape is a letter, ask the child, "What words begin with this letter?" Vary the size and color of the shapes, and ask the child to wash shapes of a specific size or color. Encourage children to squeeze using each hand individually and both hands together.

Shape Sort

Learning Reinforced

Concepts of round and square, matching, eye–hand coordination, laterality

Equipment

Small bucket of water, milk carton of water, Ping-Pong balls, square plastic blocks

Description

Ask the child to sort the round balls into the round bucket and the square blocks into the square carton. Mix the objects in both containers, and ask the child to rearrange them so they are all in the correct containers.

Variations

Increase the distance between the containers so that the child must toss the objects rather than place them. Place the container so that the child must reach across the midline of the body to reach them (shapes to the right and container to the left for right-handed children and vice versa).

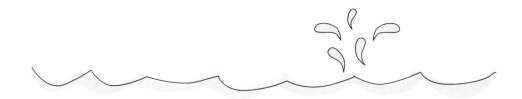

Sink the Blocks

Learning Reinforced

Concepts of floating (buoyancy), heavy and light

Equipment

Several plastic blocks, several heavier blocks that will sink, large bucket of water

Description

Place a plastic block in the water and explain *floating.* Place a heavier block in the bucket, and explain *sinking* and *weight.* Have the child hold both blocks and tell you which is heavier (or lighter). Then ask the child to place both types of blocks in the bucket, seeing which will float, which will sink, and what happens when trying to make the plastic block sink.

Variation

Try other types of objects paired as heavy and light.

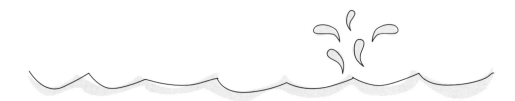

Size and Shape

Learning Reinforced

Concept of capacity, hand and arm strength and endurance, shape discrimination, size discrimination

Equipment

Foam shapes in a variety of sizes, large bucket of water, two empty containers of exactly the same size and shape

Description

Ask the child to wet two different shapes and then squeeze the water from one shape into one container and the other shape into the other container. Ask the child, "Which shape holds more water?" Try to pair large shapes with small shapes to see which shape holds more.

Variations

Compare squares, circles, triangles, rectangles, and other shapes, including letters and numbers, with each other. Ask the child to try to decide which holds more water before wringing them out and seeing the results.

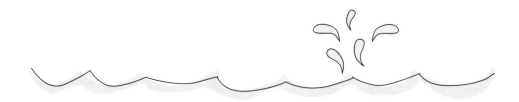

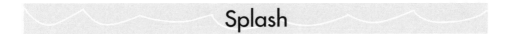

Splash

Learning Reinforced

Concepts of hard, soft, and splash; hand and arm strength and endurance; eye–hand coordination

Equipment

Large bucket of water

Description

Ask the child, "Can you make a splash?" Encourage the child to hit the top of the water with his or her hands. As the child splashes, ask him or her to hit the water *harder* or *softer* and note the different results. Splashing is fun. Be prepared to get wet!

Variations

To broaden vocabulary, substitute other terms for hard and soft (e.g., easy, gentle, powerful, forceful, big, little, large, small). To encourage creativity, ask the child to splash like a little fish, a big frog, or a happy puppy. To help improve listening, tap a rhythm on the floor with your hands. Ask the child to repeat your rhythm by hitting the surface of the water. Start with two- or three-tap rhythms and gradually increase the number of taps.

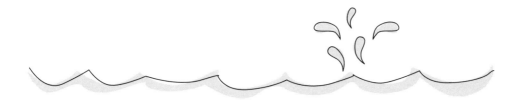

Sponge Catch

Learning Reinforced

Eye–hand coordination, hand and arm strength and endurance, grasp and release

Equipment

Several large sponges, two large buckets of water

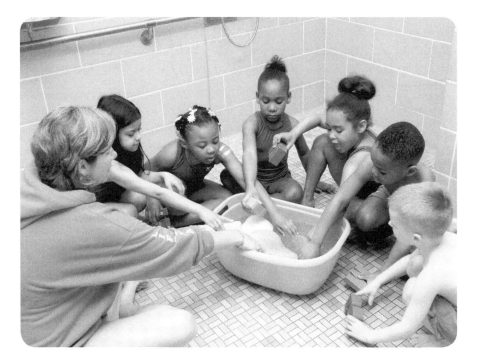

Description

Ask the child to soak a sponge in a bucket of water and then throw it to you. Catch the sponge, soak it in the bucket again, and throw it gently back to the child. Encourage the child to catch the sponge rather than just letting it land in front of him or her or letting it hit his or her body.

Variations

Vary the size and shape of the sponge for varied grasp-and-release practice. Gradually lengthen the distance between you and the child to encourage more forceful throwing.

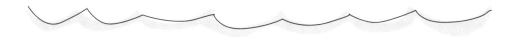

Sponge Fight

Learning Reinforced

Body-part identification, hand and arm strength and endurance, grasp and release, eye–hand coordination

Equipment

Large bucket of water, several sponges

Description

While you and a child (or two children) toss sponges at each other, ask the child to aim for specific targets (e.g., feet, legs, belly, arms). Be sure to keep the fight friendly. Praise hits that are on target: "Great throw, you got my knees wet!" Avoid terms related to actual fighting, such as *kill* and *wound*. Keep sponges dripping wet by periodically dipping them in the water. Gradually increase the distance between you and the child or the two children to encourage more forceful throwing.

Variations

Have the child throw at a target, such as an inflatable plastic figure or cardboard cutout that has been laminated to prevent water damage. Ask the child to try to hit the body parts you name. Ask the child to throw at the target and then tell you which body part the sponge hits.

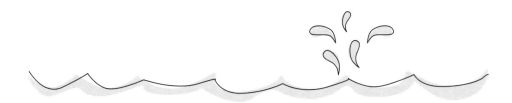

Sponge Off

Learning Reinforced

Body-part identification, hand and arm strength and endurance, eye–hand coordination

Equipment

Large bucket of water, several sponges of various textures

Description

Soak a sponge in water and rub it on different parts of the child's body. Ask the child to tell you the name of the body part as you sponge it.

Variations

Blindfold the child and ask him or her to name or wiggle the body part as you sponge it. Ask the child to sponge you to see if he or she can sponge the part you name. Vary the process further by asking the

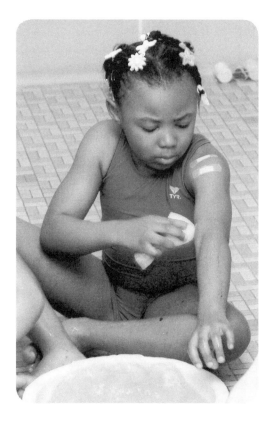

child to name a part on your body or his or her body and then sponge it. The child cannot sponge the body part if he or she cannot name it.

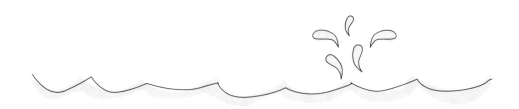

Sprinkle

Learning Reinforced

Body awareness, concept of showering, daily living activities

Equipment

Large bucket of water, watering can

Description

Fill the watering can with water and sprinkle each child. Talk about what a shower or being out in the rain is like. Sprinkle a part of the child's body. Ask the child, "What part of you am I sprinkling?" You can combine this with a cleanup activity or a body-part identification activity.

Variations

Ask the child to name and sprinkle parts of your body, naming a different part with each sprinkle. After the child is familiar with the activity, add a blindfold and ask the child to feel which part of the body you are sprinkling.

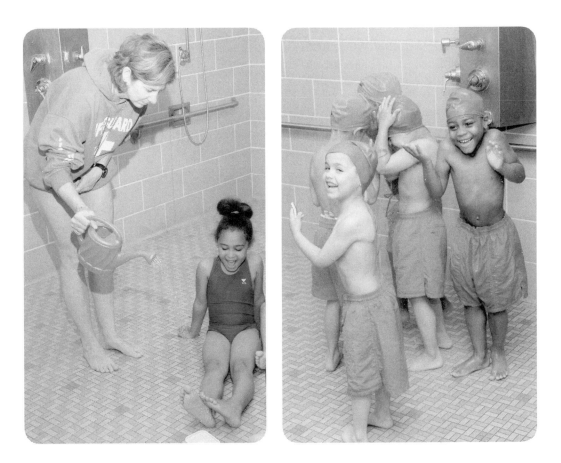

Squeeze

Learning Reinforced

Hand and arm strength and endurance, grasp and squeeze

Equipment

Empty squeeze bottle (e.g., mustard or small dish-soap bottle) containers with openings in a variety of sizes, large bucket of water

Description

Fill the squeeze bottle and have the child use it to fill the empty containers. The child ejects water by squeezing the bottle. Encourage the child to use one hand at a time and both hands together. Gradually work from a container with a large mouth to one with a small one. Also, gradually lengthen the distance

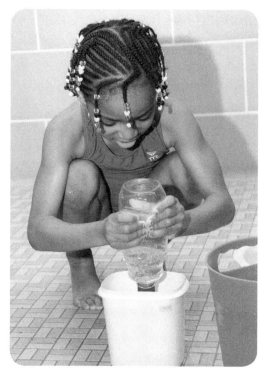

between the child and the container. You can also use the squeeze bottle to fill the bucket and use it in a variety of body awareness and body-part identification activities.

Variations

Vary the size of the squeeze bottle. Substitute a squeeze container for the Pour and Fill activity or Scoop and Fill activity (see pages 63 and 66, respectively).

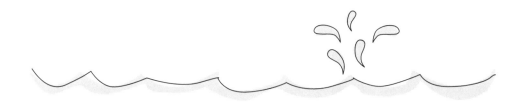

Squirt and Fill

Learning Reinforced

Hand and arm strength and endurance, finger dexterity, concept of capacity, eye–hand coordination, grasp and squeeze

Equipment

Squirt gun or squeeze bottle, large bucket of water, empty containers with openings in a variety of sizes

Description

Ask the child to fill the squirt gun from the bucket, and then ask "Can you use your squirt gun to fill the empty containers?" Gradually work from a container with a large mouth to one with a small one. Also, gradually lengthen the distance from the gun to the container.

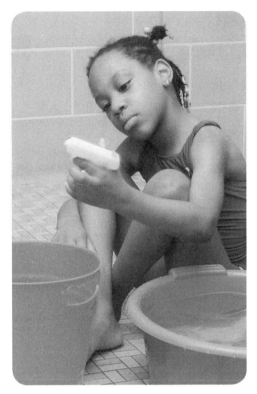

Variations

Ask the child to fill the container half full (three-quarters full, more than half full, a quarter full). Ask the child to see how fast he or she can repeatedly squirt (avoid saying "pull the trigger"). Count out loud how many squirts it takes to fill a small container. On subsequent days see if the child can better his or her time. For increased difficulty, ask the child, "How many squirts do you think it will take to fill this container?"

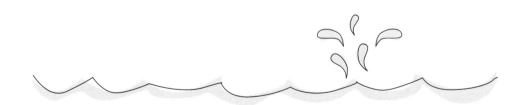

Squirt Guns

Learning Reinforced

Hand and arm strength and endurance, finger dexterity, eye–hand coordination, grasp and squeeze

Equipment

Large bucket of water, squirt gun, colored construction paper targets

Description

Ask the child to fill the squirt gun from the bucket and then squirt at the paper target. It may be necessary to experiment to find the best distance from the child to the target.

Variation

Use pictures of different things for targets and ask the child to name the color or part of the picture that he or she hits. This activity does not have to simulate hunting; instead, make targets of different flowers and water the flowers.

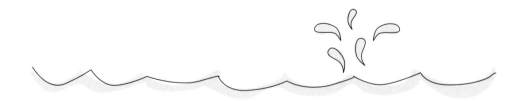

Squirt Your Body

Learning Reinforced

Body-part identification, hand and arm strength and endurance, finger dexterity, eye–hand coordination, grasp and squeeze

Equipment

Squirt gun, bucket of water

Description

Ask the child to fill the gun from the large bucket of water. Then ask, "Can you squirt a part of your body while naming that part?"

Variations

Squirt different parts and ask the child to name them. To challenge different senses, blindfold the child and ask him or her to name the parts you squirt or to wiggle them.

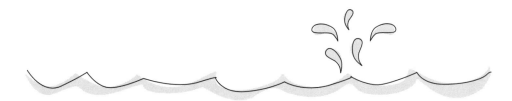

Stacking

Learning Reinforced

Finger dexterity, concepts of floating and size

Equipment

A stacking toy (plastic base with center dowel on which plastic rings are stacked), large bucket of water

Description

Place the base of the stacking toy, without the rings on it, into the bucket. Ask the child to stack the rings appropriately onto the base (usually this is big first, tapering to small). Through experimentation, the child should find and hold down the base. The child must hold down the rings as he or she stacks them, otherwise they float off. It is also necessary to stack the rings according to size. It might be helpful for the child to try the toy out of the bucket first to increase his or her understanding of the task.

Variations

Ask the child to name the colors and sizes as he or she stacks. Ask the child to count the rings as he or she stacks them.

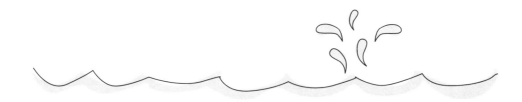

Take Out

Learning Reinforced

Finger dexterity; concepts of find, take, and put; object identification

Equipment

Large bucket of water, a variety of objects (some that float and some that sink)

Description

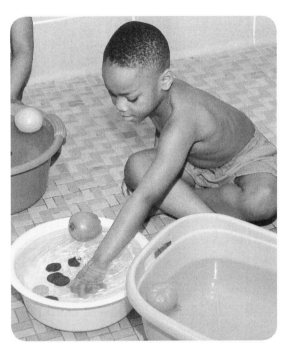

Place all the objects in the bucket. Name an object and ask the child to find it, take it out of the bucket, and put it next to him or her. Once the child has taken out several objects, add the command to put objects in the bucket and then mix the commands so that objects go in both directions.

Variations

Substitute a picture of the object for the name. Ask the child, "Can you find something that matches this?" Omit the object's name from your request. Ask the child, "What is this?" Blindfold the child and ask him or her to identify the object you name by its shape and texture. If the match is correct, reinforce and praise the child by saying, "Yes, you found the _____. Good job!"

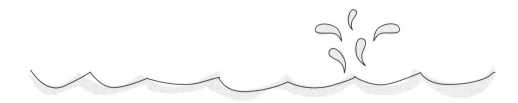

Underwater Puzzles

Learning Reinforced

Finger dexterity, visual perception, object permanence

Equipment

Wooden-framed puzzle, tub of water big enough that the puzzle frame can lie flat on the bottom (To make a wooden puzzle water resistant, varnish each piece with marine varnish.)

Description

Show the child the finished puzzle. Then, take it apart and put the frame and puzzle parts into the tub. Ask the child, "Can you put this back together again?"

Variations

Start with puzzles that have large pieces. Progress to smaller piece sizes and more complex puzzle pictures.

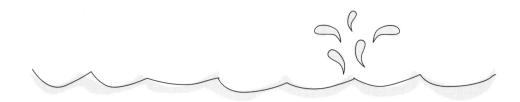

Washcloth Substitute

Learning Reinforced
Varies

Equipment
Washcloth, variety of other items

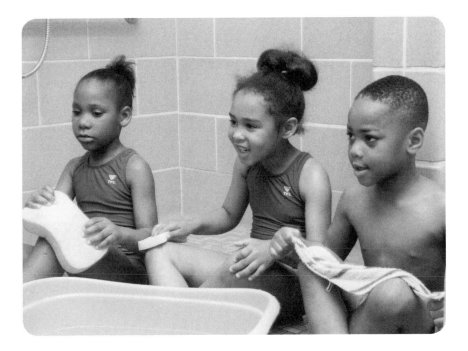

Description
Substitute a washcloth or other absorbent item in any activity that uses a sponge.

Variations
Use washcloths of various colors and ask the child to match them with objects of the same color. To vary the weight during the task, use washcloths of different sizes. Use washcloths of different textures for activities involving contact with various body parts.

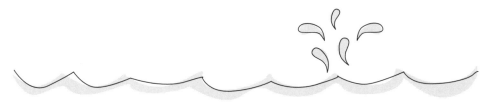

Water Body Painting

Learning Reinforced

Body awareness, body-part identification, kinesthetic awareness

Equipment

Paintbrushes, small bucket of water

Description

Ask the child to use a wet brush and paint different body parts with water and name the part as he or she paints it. Have the child wiggle the part as you or the child paints it.

Variation

Blindfold the child and ask him or her to name or wiggle the part as it is painted.

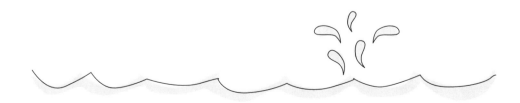

Water Sidewalk and Wall Painting

Learning Reinforced

Hand and arm strength and endurance, finger dexterity, printing, eye–hand coordination

Equipment

Paintbrushes of various sizes, several buckets of water, sidewalk or wall surface on which water will leave a mark (If using a wall, select a waterproof wall, and tape construction paper to it to create a porous surface that will show the water mark. **Note:** Paint with clear water so that it leaves no mark when it dries.)

Description

Ask the child to use a brush wet with water to paint the wall or sidewalk. Let the child practice making letters, numerals, faces, or objects.

Variations

Paint outlines, and ask the child to fill them in. Paint shapes and objects and ask the child to guess what they are. Paint a figure, then ask the child, "Can you copy my drawing?" Paint shadows.

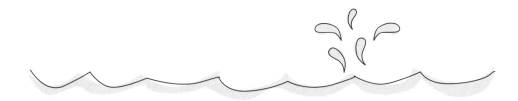

Water Soap Bubbles

Learning Reinforced
Breath control, blowing

Equipment
Large bucket of water, straws, liquid soap

Description
When the child can success-fully accomplish the Blow activity (see page 41) using a straw—avoids sucking water in—add liquid soap to the water. Ask the child to blow with a straw to see if he or she can make big bubbles. Seeing bubbles that are big encourages blowing.

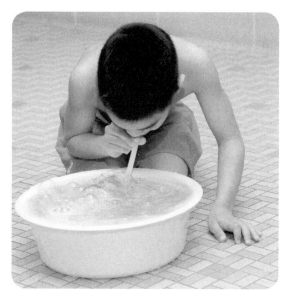

Variation
Add food color to the water to change the color of the bubbles.

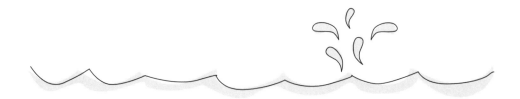

Water Talking

Learning Reinforced
Breath control

Equipment
Large tub of water

Description
When the child can successfully and consistently do Face Dunks and Face Dunks and Bubbles (see pages 49 and 50), has relatively good breath control, and can put his or her entire face in the water without drinking or inhaling water, ask the child to say his or her name or other familiar words underwater.

Variation
Place a laminated flash card in the water without showing it to the child first. The card could have a word, number, or picture on it. Ask the child, "Can you put your face in, look at the card, and while your face is still underwater tell me what is on the card?" What the child says will be difficult to understand, but that is half the fun. Ask the child to repeat the word when he or she lifts his or her face out of the water.

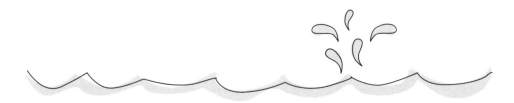

Wet and Heavy

Learning Reinforced
Concepts of heavy and light

Equipment
Foam shapes, sponges or washcloths, large bucket of water

Description
Ask the child to hold a dry object in one hand and a wet one in the other and ask, "Which object is heavier? Which object weighs less?" It should be fairly easy for the child to feel the difference, and in most cases the wet object will be heavier.

Variations
Use objects of various sizes so that the wet object is not always the heaviest. Increase the difficulty of the task by selecting objects that will challenge the child's ability to judge weight. For example, a dry rock and a wet plastic block will be different from a wet wash-cloth and a dry plastic block.

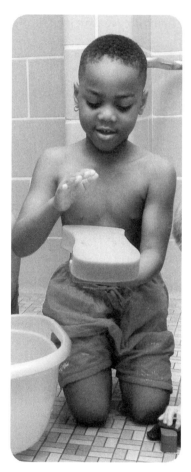

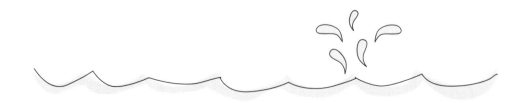

Wring Out

Learning Reinforced

Hand and arm strength and endurance, grasp and squeeze

Equipment

Washcloth, large bucket of water

Description

Ask the child, "Can you get the washcloth all wet?" Then ask, "Can you squeeze all the water out of the washcloth?"

Variations

Ask the child to fill an empty container when wringing out the cloth. Gradually increase the size of the cloth and demonstrate actual wringing (as compared to squeezing) to encourage using both hands together.

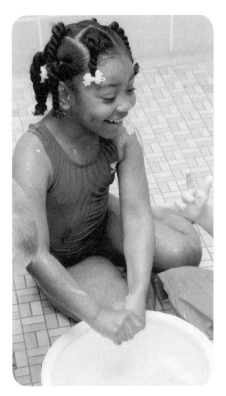

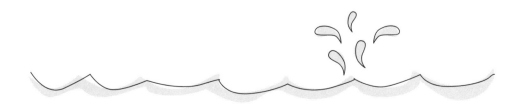

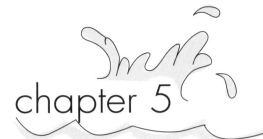

chapter 5

Water Learning Activities for the Pool Environment

Planning a water learning activity session for the pool begins by determining the goals for 6-year-old Samantha. She is working on improving balance and spatial orientation. Samantha is in first grade, reading easy books, and doing addition and subtraction. Her writing skills need improvement. Because Samantha has a slight learning disability she also participates in a recreation therapy program to help her keep up with her peers. To help Samantha improve in the selected areas, Samantha's facilitator in the recreation therapy program looks at the learning reinforced column in the activity finder and, based on Samantha's needs, chooses Movement Exploration, Poly Trail, Statue, and Musical Spots for the day's session.

The recreation therapy program takes place at the local community pool where Samantha participates with several other children. While the group is getting dressed, the group facilitator, already in his swimsuit, scatters poly spots on the bottom of the pool in the shallow end. A pool lifeguard supervises.

For the next 30 minutes, Samantha and the other children in her group solve movement problems set by her facilitator. He asks the following questions:

Can you move around our space without stepping on any spots?

Can you move faster? Even faster? Slower? Even slower? Very slowly?

Note: The progression is from any speed of movement to a more controlled movement speed.

Can you move by stepping from spot to spot?

Note: The progression is toward specific foot placement.

Now we are going to play Statue. Can you move without stepping on a spot until you hear me say statue? When you hear me say statue, stand on the nearest spot and make a statue.

Note: The children must not only move without touching spots but also move on a cue, change to stepping on a spot, and then control their action to remain still.

Let's add music! When the music starts, can you move from spot to spot, and when the music stops, can you make a statue?

Note: Adding musical cues increases the difficulty of the progression because children must remember what to do when they hear the musical cue. The cue does not, in and of itself, tell them.

The session isn't over yet. Now that the children have participated in active learning through the movement sequences, the facilitator changes to the Poly Trail activity and rearranges the spots on the bottom of the pool. Because these children have all been diagnosed with ADHD, their facilitator has saved this task for after the music-and-movement activity, recognizing that Samantha and the other children will do better if they spend pent-up energy before needing to concentrate.

Finally, Samantha and her facilitator try some of the activities from the previous water learning session. On the Spot was a favorite. **Note:** At the end of the session, return to an easier task and one that is fun to be sure to end on a positive note.

At the end of the session, Samantha and the other children head for the locker room, and the facilitator makes notes to document progress, to aid in planning for the next session, and for the children to take home to their parents.

Big Boat

A big boat can be any large platform or container used for balance activities. The big boat pictured in this chapter is available from Aquam (Champlain, New York, www.aquam.com). Activities using the big boat can help improve and assess motor planning, balance, strength, flexibility, color recognition, math skills, the ability to grasp and release, and the ability to follow directions. During activities, you can use the big boat empty or filled with plastic balls.

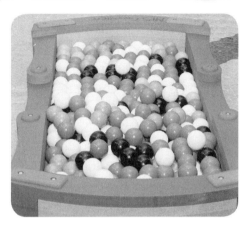

Color Object Sort

Learning Reinforced
Color recognition, grasp and release, matching, sorting

Equipment
Variety of colored objects, mesh bags in same colors as objects, big boat

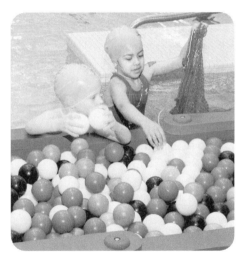

Description
Place the objects in the boat. Give the child a mesh bag and ask, "Can you fill your bag with objects that match the color of the bag?" The floating movement of the big boat makes grasping and releasing more difficult. If the child puts objects in the bag that do not match, remove them, hold them next to the bag, and ask the child, "Does this object match this bag?" If the child answers yes, correct the child by saying, "No, these do not match. This object is one that matches." Then show the child an object that is the correct color and try the activity again.

Variation
Select objects that vary in size and shape to increase the difficulty of the task.

Boat Crawl

Learning Reinforced

Balance, body image, strength, flexibility, motor planning

Equipment

Big boat, plastic balls (Filling the boat with small plastic balls increases the difficulty because both the boat and the balls will move.)

Description

Position the child on one side of the big boat and ask, "Can you move across the boat to the other side?" Hold the boat to provide stability as the child moves across. Allow gentle rocking as his or her balance improves.

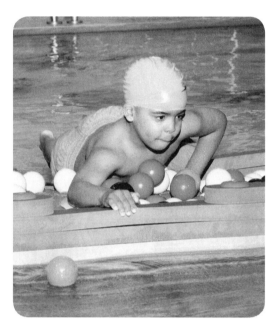

Safety Tips

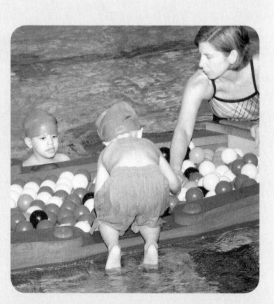

- Using the term *move* allows the child to cross in any manner. Some children may decide to try to stand in the boat, so be sure the boat is in water deep enough that if the child stands and falls, there is no risk of spinal injury. When working with small children, the water level should be at the child's chest, and you should encourage the child to enter the water feet first.

- Asking the child, "Can you come off feet first?" facilitates safety by teaching a feet-first entry into the water. It also requires additional motor planning by the child.

Boat Statue

Learning Reinforced
Balance, body image, strength, flexibility

Equipment
Big boat, plastic balls (Filling the boat with small plastic balls increases the difficulty because both the boat and the balls will move.)

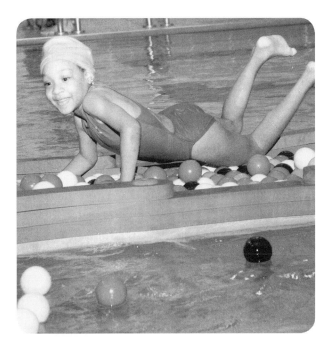

Description
Ask the child, "Can you get on top of the boat?" Once the child is there, ask him or her to "freeze" and make a statue. Start by asking, "Can you freeze while I count to three?" Gradually increase the length of time the child must balance.

Variations
Ask the child to move around on the big boat and become still like a statue whenever you say freeze. Time your freeze challenges so that the child must hold his or her balance in various positions. It adds to the challenge if you ask the child to make a specific type of statue. For example, ask, "Can you make a scary statue?" or "Can you make a statue of a puppy?"

Clothing

Asking a child to wear clothing in addition to a bathing suit while in the pool can be especially useful in helping a child develop body image and improve balance. The additional weight of wet clothing increases awareness of the parts of the body carrying this additional weight. Clothing weight also acts as an anchor by decreasing buoyancy and helps a child become more aware of the bottom of the pool. This will help improve balance and mobility. Performing water learning activities while wearing clothes helps increase strength as muscles work to move the additional weight.

Wet Dressing

Learning Reinforced

Dressing and undressing, balance, body image, finger dexterity, strength, flexibility

Equipment

A variety of clean clothing (Start with short trousers and a short-sleeved T-shirt one size larger than the child usually wears. This makes the initial task easier. Gradually progress to long trousers and a long-sleeved shirt in the child's size. Heavier fabric increases the challenge.)

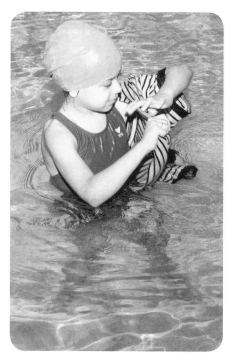

Description

The child begins on land, putting on the trousers and shirt over his or her swimsuit. Then, he or she enters the water. After the child moves around to get used to being dressed and totally wet, ask the child, "Can you take off your shirt? Can you take off your trousers?" Once the trousers and shirt have been removed, ask the child, "Can you put the wet clothes back on?"

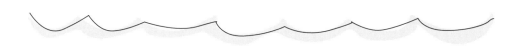

Variations

Ask the child if he or she can stand on a poly spot and remove the clothing items. Add clean tennis shoes to the attire, and then ask the child, "Which would you like to take off first?" or "Which is the heaviest item of clothing?" This requires the child to use kinesthetic feedback to assess weight and teaches the water safety concept of taking off the heaviest item first in an emergency. This activity can also be done in a nonpool water learning environment.

Safety Tip

As the child removes a pullover shirt, provide assistance to be sure that the child's head does not get stuck in the shirt. This could cause fear and could inhibit breathing.

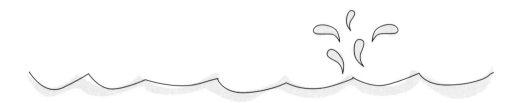

Cone Academics

Traffic cones come in a variety of sizes and colors. The tops of some cones are made with a small slit into which a card can be inserted. Other cones, shown here, come with letters and numbers that fit over the top.

These cones provide a variety of opportunities for integrating reading (signs and letters), math, and other academic tasks with water activities. Laminated cards can show objects, activities, and academic challenges.

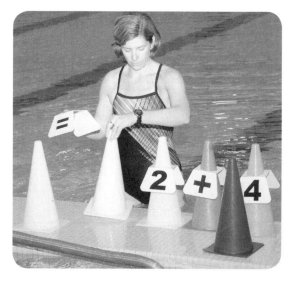

Circuit Training

Learning Reinforced

Physical fitness, imitation, reading signs, counting

Equipment

Six cones and six activity cards, each showing a child performing a different exercise

Description

Place the cone and card combinations along the side of the pool. Ask the child, "Can you visit each cone and perform the activity you see on the card?" If your goal is greater orientation to water, cards can depict beginner swim skills. If repetitions are specified on the card, ask the child to count out loud as he or she completes the repetitions.

Variation

For increased cardiorespiratory fitness, the child can perform the circuit for time, jogging from card to card, trying to improve the time over his or her last performance.

Cone Matching

Learning Reinforced
Matching, object retrieval

Equipment
One cone, a variety of sinkable objects with matching cards (Scatter the objects on the pool bottom.)

Description
Place a card in the cone. Ask the child, "Can you look at the card and then find something on the bottom of the pool that matches what you see on the card?" When the child returns with the object, hold it next to the card and ask the child, "Do they match?" (thus having the child solve another problem independently).

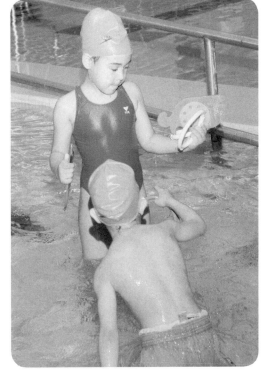

Variations
Use cards showing activities of daily living and the objects needed to perform the tasks (e.g., brushing teeth and a tooth brush, combing hair and a comb). Matching by function as well as by picture reinforces academic learning. Use cards of different colors for a color match. Use number cards, and ask the child, "Can you find this many objects?"

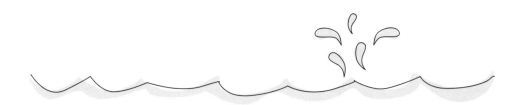

Cone Math

Learning Reinforced

Number recognition, math

Equipment

Cones, cards with a variety of math problems, random collection of sinkable objects

Description

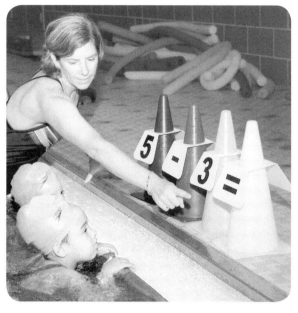

Scatter objects on the bottom of the pool, and then place a math card on the cone or a series of cards on several cones. Ask the child, "Can you pick up enough objects to solve this problem?" (Allow the child to choose his or her retrieval method and the level of submersion he or she is comfortable with.) Problems might include the following:

- The child retrieves the number of objects shown on a card.
- The child retrieves the number of objects equal to the answer of an addition, subtraction, multiplication, or division problem.
- The child retrieves objects in groups in order to manually work out the problem. For example, to solve an addition problem, ask the child to retrieve objects to match the first number in the equation. Then ask the child to retrieve objects to match the second number. Finally, ask the child to count all of the objects to obtain the total.

Variations

Set up a cone trail consisting of several cones with different problems. Ask the child to move from cone to cone, solving problems at each cone. Increase the difficulty by timing how long it takes the child to solve all problems on the trail. Change the numbers in the problems (but do not increase the overall difficulty) and time the child again, encouraging the child to proceed more quickly through the new trail. Increased speed in moving along the trail and retrieving objects will increase fitness and breath control. Increased speed in solving the math problems will improve mental processing.

Interpretive Movement

I'm just a little kitten. I'm tiny and gray with white paws.

I'm furry, and I love to **wiggle.**

Sometimes, when I first wake up, I have to **stretch.**

I **reach** up high with both my paws.

Then I have to **stretch** my claws.

I love to **climb** all around my yard. No high tree is too difficult.

I **jump** over the hose.

I **leap** to chase a butterfly.

I **race** to catch the bunny when he comes around our garden.

I even practice my kitten **roar.**

The backyard is my favorite place to **play**

and, frankly, where I'd rather stay.

Franklin is a wonderful kitten story. It has a main character that children can relate to. Franklin does lots of things and has fun while being active. During water learning, children can act out the story of Franklin, pretending they are this happy, active kitten. Just think of all the things Franklin (and the children) can do. Franklin's story becomes water learning when the facilitator tells the story and asks the children to pretend they are Franklin.

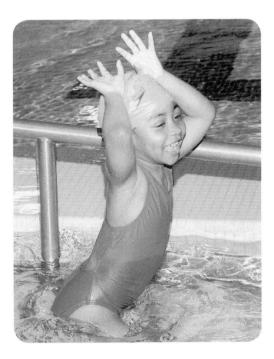

This is interpretive movement in the pool.

- What types of stories work best for interpretive movement? Stories with actions that children can imitate, for example, *The Little Engine That Could,* are appropriate. So are stories with characters that children already know and associate with movements or activities, such as *Peter Pan* (who flies). Hero stories, such as Harry Potter playing Quidditch, are well suited for interpretive movement. These could be contemporary, fictional, or historical.

- Where do you find the stories? A bookstore or library might get you started, but the very best stories are right in your own imagination. Franklin exists nowhere else, not in print or video or song. He's a brand new kitten. You too can create a Franklin or a Puff or a Twiddlelumpkin or a Salibewicket. Children will love your characters; add movements to your characters and give them life.

Build into your story the movements you feel a child should work on: locomotor patterns, flexibility stretches, continuous repetitions to build endurance, ongoing activity to emphasize cardiorespiratory fitness, complicated obstacles to focus on spatial orientation. You can build into an interpretive movement activity any learning you want to reinforce.

You might want to plan stories that include pictures. Laminating keeps a picture from being damaged by water. You can also laminate small books. Having pictures available to stimulate the creative process is helpful for children who are visual, rather than auditory, learners. Colored pictures gain attention more quickly than black and white pictures. Action pictures spur the viewer into action.

Lion Hunt

Learning Reinforced

Imitation, flexibility, endurance, cardiorespiratory fitness, laterality, directionality, spatial orientation, creativity

Equipment

None

Description

Lion Hunt is an activity with a facilitator and child followers. The facilitator takes the followers on a lion hunt. As the facilitator tells the lion hunt story, he or she leads an action for each part of the story. The facilitator asks the children to imitate joining in the hunt. Here is a typical Lion Hunt story, with facilitator actions included in parentheses.

Let's go on a lion hunt!

We need to pick up our pack (pantomime putting on backpack).

Let's start walking (walk in place, swinging arms).

We have a long hike; let's walk a little faster (pick up the pace).

Wow, this grass is sure tall. Let's push it out of our way
(reach forward with both hands and push water out to each side).

Look at this big log. We have to step over it
(take large, high step over imaginary log).

Good job! Wow, the weather is great for a lion hunt, let's jog a little (jog).

I hear a lion roar (stop, tilt head, bring hand to ear to listen).

It sounds like a big lion. Let's go find it (start walking quickly).

Here's a tree. Let's climb to the top to see if we can see the lion
(simulate tree climbing with arms and legs).

Where is that lion (hold imaginary tree with one arm,
put other hand at eyebrow and search for lion)?

There he is! Let's swing down and find him
(grasp imaginary vine and swing to ground and start running).

Aggh! He is coming this way. Help
(stop, freeze, point, and run fast in the opposite direction)!

I'm scared of lions (run faster).

Whew! It is good to be back home
(big sigh, stop running, relax, and shake out).

Great lion hunt, everyone!

(continued)

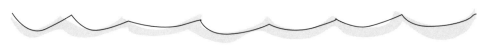

(continued)

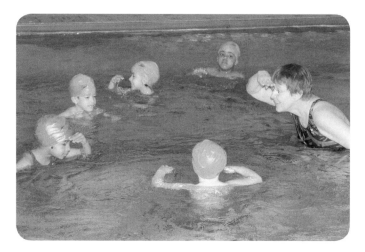

When planning a Lion Hunt activity story, keep in mind the developmental goals for the child, and select story components to help meet these goals. For example, if a child needs to improve endurance or cardiorespiratory fitness, build in a lot of continuous walking, jogging, and running actions with accompanying arm actions. If a child needs to improve the extension of one or both arms, build in activities that use the arms to repeatedly reach and pull. If a child needs to improve hip flexibility, include stepping over large objects, taking giant steps, walking in mud or quicksand, or running through snowdrifts.

Variations

Use any action story appropriate for the age and interest of the child. Celebrate holidays. You can explore a haunted house, help Santa deliver presents, or be in the Fourth of July parade. Ask the child to be the storyteller, relating his or her story to you, including actions of his or her choosing. Follow along and imitate the actions of the child as he or she takes you into his or her magical world.

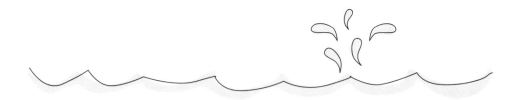

Jobs

In a school setting, learning is all about task completion. Daily, children hear "Finish your assignment," "Finish your project," "Finish your lunch," "Finish . . ." Presenting activities as tasks to complete—jobs—helps reinforce this important educational theme.

Undertaking and completing a job also introduces children to the world of work by helping them develop responsibility for accomplishment. Combined with success and praise, jobs help build self-confidence and self-esteem. A child can be proud of a job well done.

A job can reinforce any aspect of learning. The locomotor pattern used to accomplish the job can reinforce any motor skill. The obstacles you place in the path of children completing the jobs can challenge many different facets of perceptual-motor development.

In structuring a job for completion, you can say to a single child, in a manner much like you would in any other problem-solving activity, "Here is your job. Can you _____? When you are finished with your job, come back to me."

A group of children will need more structure. When working with a group, designate a starting and finishing place. At the starting place you will give the children the specifics of the job. They will return to the finishing place with their completed work. Provide a start and finish signal. Include the parameters of safe participation, for example, remind children to walk on a ramp.

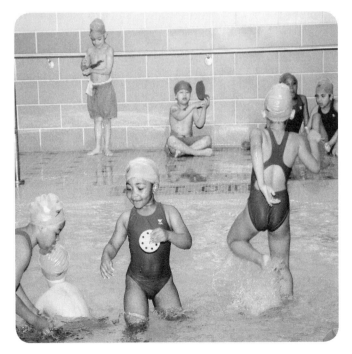

Color Match

Learning Reinforced

Color recognition, matching, grasp and release, object retrieval

Equipment

Colored paper, sinkable objects in colors matching the paper

Description

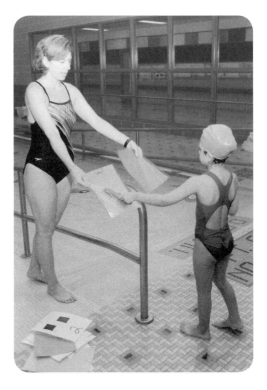

Scatter the objects in the water. Ask the children to perform the job of finding an object that matches the color of the paper you are holding. If children are on the pool deck, provide reminders on safe pool entry. Tell them when they have completed their job to return to the starting point. Signal them to begin their work. For example, "This is green. Your job is to find a green object. Can you find a green object? Be sure to slide in feet first. Bring your green object back to me. Ready, begin your job."

Notice, the starting signal is "Begin your job." This reinforces the job aspect of the task. Using go as a starting signal turns the activity into a race ("ready, set, go!"). Because job performance usually is not a race, avoid using race cues. As children return to the start position, have the colored paper available so they can be sure they are correct. When a child returns to the start, ask the name of the color he or she found. Praise good work. "You did good work finishing that job!" For the next color, ask the children to put the color they have back into the water (place, not throw) and bring back an object to match the new color.

Variations

Show more than one color at the start. Working from retrieving one color to retrieving two, then three, and then four colors makes the task progressively more difficult. Increase the depth of the water where objects are placed, being careful the depth does not exceed the child's swimming ability. For children who cannot swim, place objects in water no higher than the child's chest.

Sink or Float?

Learning Reinforced

Concept of floating (buoyancy), grasp and release, object retrieval, matching

Equipment

Two signs (one picturing waves and an object on top of the waves, labeled float, and one picturing waves and an object on the bottom of the sign, labeled sink), a variety of objects that sink, a variety of objects that float

Description

Scatter the objects in the pool. Show students both signs and explain the difference between float and sink and why floating is important for learning to swim. Then show either the float picture or the sink picture, but do not name the action. Ask the children to find objects like the picture you show them. Say to the children, "Your job is

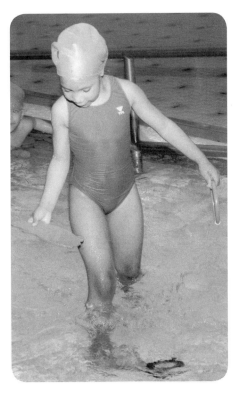

to find objects that do this. Can you find objects that do this? Find one and bring it back here to me."

When children return, allow them to match the action of the object they find with what they see on the picture. They can either match the picture or read the word. If a child brings back an incorrect object, show the child what that object does when you place it in the water. Ask the child, "Does this float or sink?" Clarify incorrect information by saying, "It looks like this doesn't ____. It _____." Then try the job again.

Variations

Add number concepts to increase the difficulty by asking the child to retrieve a specific number of objects or asking for a specific number of objects that sink and a specific number of objects that float. Ask for objects of specific colors, alone or in combination with numbers and buoyancy.

What's What?

Learning Reinforced

Matching, object identification, grasp and release

Equipment

Objects that sink and objects that float, pictures of people using similar objects

Description

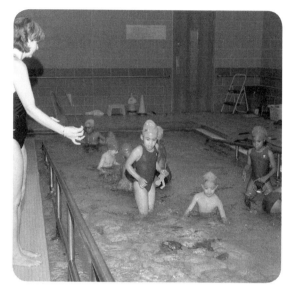

Scatter the objects in the pool. Show the child a picture of a person using one of the objects. For example, if one of the objects is a comb, show the child a picture of a person combing his or her hair. Ask the child, "What object is this person using? Your job is to find the same object. Can you find a comb?" When the child returns with the correct object, praise the child, "Yes, you did a good job. That is a comb." Then discuss what a comb is used for. If the child retrieves an incorrect object, compare the incorrect object with the picture and discuss why this isn't a match. Repeat the job. When moving on to the next object, have the child return the object to the pool when beginning the search for the new object.

Variations

Increase the number of objects the child should find. For example, if the picture is of someone drinking cocoa, ask the child to retrieve the cup and saucer. For greater difficulty, omit pictures, and provide only verbal clues. For example, if you want the child to find a comb, don't show a picture, but instead, say, "Can you find a comb?" Even greater difficulty results if you do not name the object but rather ask for it by function. "Your job is to find what you use to make your hair neat and tidy. Can you find something to do that?"

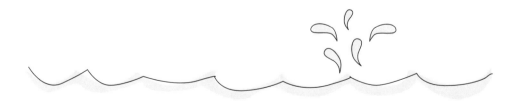

Count, Add, and Subtract

Learning Reinforced

Math concepts, matching, counting

Equipment

A variety of objects that sink, a variety of objects that float, cards with dots and numbers

Description

Hold up one card. Ask the children to determine the number of dots on the card or identify the number and find that many objects. Initially, use one card with one to six dots. Marking your card like dice will help children who play board games that use dice. Gradually include additional cards to work with higher numbers.

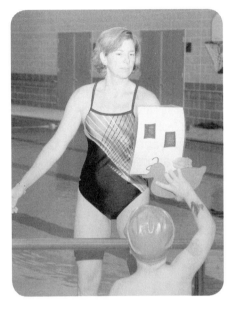

Variations

Ask children to add the numbers on two cards and bring back that many objects. Explore math processes (addition, subtraction, multiplication, and division) by placing math symbols between two cards with dots. Create cards of different colors. Make the dots on one card one color and the dots on other cards other colors. When selecting objects, the child must not only accumulate the appropriate number of objects but also objects of the correct color. To further increase the difficulty, make the dots different sizes—small and large. In this variation, children must bring back objects of the appropriate size and color. And the quantity must match the number or the solution to the math problem.

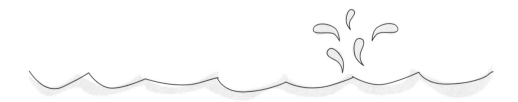

Movement Exploration

Movement exploration allows children to explore their immediate environment at their own pace and at a comfortable level of engagement. Facilitated by a problem-solving, questioning technique, movement exploration can focus on any motor pattern or movement quality. To establish an environment appropriate for freedom of movement, tell the children they can move wherever they want to, provided they stay within the stated boundaries. Then, state the boundaries. For example, "We are going to move around our space. You can go anywhere you want, as long as you stay in the pool, off the steps, and on this side of the lifeline." Remind children to be careful not to touch another person while moving. Say "Remember to share our space, and be careful not to touch anyone else." Once children are moving, you will ask questions, which they should answer with movement. In movement exploration, there is no right or wrong response, just levels of engagement. Be sure to praise engaged responses. Ask additional questions to refine movement quality.

Movement Basics

Learning Reinforced

Locomotion in water; directionality; spatial orientation; concepts of speed, distance, and height; cardiorespiratory fitness; endurance; creativity

Equipment

None

Description

Ask the children to find their space in the water. Explain that this is their personal space and they should not be able to touch anyone else or to touch the side of the pool, ladder, and so on.

Once everyone has a space, ask problem-solving questions that will stimulate movement. The following are examples:

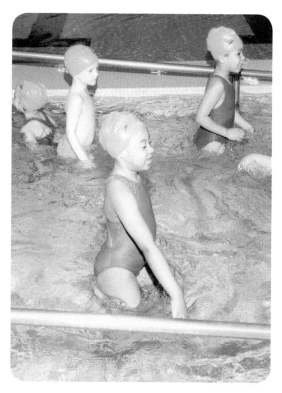

- Can you move all around our water space?
- Can you move without bumping or splashing anyone else?
- Can you move faster? Even faster? Even faster? Slower? Very slowly? Very, very slowly?
- Can you move forward (or backward or sideward)?
- Can you move in circles? In circles and forward (or backward) at the same time?
- Can you bounce? Can you bounce and move forward (or backward or sideward)?
- Can you make bigger bounces? Even bigger bounces? How high can you bounce? Can you touch the ceiling (or sky)?
- Can you spin while you move?
- Can you tiptoe? Can you tiptoe with tiny steps?

You can add any movement pattern to the movement sequence, gradually adding combinations and qualifiers as children become more mobile. The longer the movement continues, the greater the potential for developing cardiorespiratory fitness and endurance. When working with a group of children, no two responses will be the same. Movement exploration fosters individual creativity. Provide feedback while a child is moving to reinforce effort.

- That's really high. Can you go higher?
- Good job on taking big steps.
- Wonderful moving without touching anyone!
- You got really close to the bottom.

Variations

Add specific examples to the movement challenges to help children explore the movement of common objects and animals. For example, ask, "Can you move around our space like a duck? Can you move around like a race car? Can you fly around our space like a jet?" Don't forget the imagination. Ask, "Can you move around our space like a sprackity whatchet?" or "Can you make magic sparks while you fly around on your magic carpet?"

Enhanced Movement Exploration

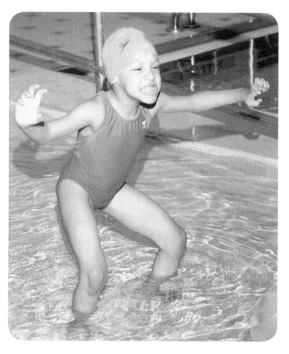

Learning Reinforced

Body image, balance, laterality, directionality, spatial orientation, endurance, cardio-respiratory fitness, creativity

Equipment

A variety of objects that float and objects that sink

Description

Adding equipment increases the difficulty of movement exploration and working with objects of different sizes, whether they float or sink, and objects of several different colors can increase a child's problem-solving abilities. The child uses the same problem-solving techniques he or she used in Movement Basics but must meet additional challenges. These challenges might include the following:

- Place a variety of floating objects inside the movement area and ask the children, "Can you move around without touching any of the floating objects?"

- Place a variety of sinkable objects on the pool bottom. Ask the children, "Can you move around without touching any of the submerged objects?"

- Place a variety of floating and submerged objects in the movement area and ask the children, "Can you move around without touching any of the objects?"

- As the children move around, place floating objects in front of them unexpectedly to force a spur-of-the-moment change in direction to avoid touching them.

- As the children move around, place a variety of objects in their path.

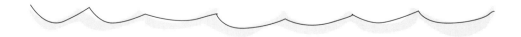

Ask them, "Can you move backward when you come to something yellow? Can you change direction when you come to something red? Can you spin in a circle when you come to something blue?"

- To create the more difficult challenge of submersion, ask, "Can you go under each floating object you come to?"

Variation

In all of the described challenges, the more fantasy you can weave into the directions, the more fun the activity will be for the children. Avoiding "sharks" (the objects on the bottom), moving around "traps" (floating objects), and ducking away from the falling "poison arrows" (objects you launch into each child's path) also challenge the imagination.

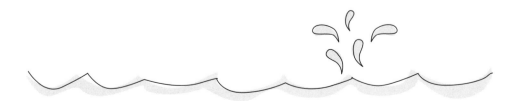

Musical Activities

Music makes most land activities more fun. The same can be said for adding music to water learning activities in the pool. However, when deciding whether to use music in a pool setting, you must consider the noise level already present, the quality of the sound system you will use, and the auditory-arousal level of the child. In an already noisy pool, adding music can result in auditory overload in children with problems in auditory perception. For children with visual disabilities, music may interfere with their ability to hear the environmental sounds necessary for spatial orientation. Additional auditory input can cause hyperactivity or emotional stress in a child who is easily overstimulated. If the sound system can produce a clear sound and you can control the decibel level and participants are comfortable with the music, music can broaden water learning opportunities. Your music selection depends on the activity goals. Music designed to enhance movement experiences is a good place to start. This includes recordings that contain the following:

- Cues for exercises (jumping jacks, jogging, and so on) and accompanying music to stimulate activity
- Movement exploration narratives that establish situations in which children "move until the music stops, then freeze" or "hop, skip, run, jump" as different types of music provide cues
- Dance stories or narrated stories, with accompanying music, that children act out
- Sing-along songs that include lyrics with physical actions, such as "She'll Be Coming 'Round the Mountain"
- Dance music for square dance, line dance, polka, and other dance forms, which can be done in the pool, with just a little additional planning (Grosse 2005)

Using music with vocal directions allows facilitators the freedom to dance with the children. This makes everyone a participant rather than just child participants dancing with other children. Sometimes it is easier for a child to develop social skills when playing with a facilitator, whose behavior is always appropriate and full of praise and good social cueing. Once a child has tried out a social skill and been successful (or been helpfully corrected), the child will be more confident playing with other children. There are even CDs and cassettes specifically prepared for water learning, such as the Learning Station's *Sift and Splash,* available from Wagon Wheel Records, Huntington Beach, California (www.wagonwheelrecords.net).

Noodles

Long, colorful, and made of foam, noodles have a variety of uses in water learning. They are easy for children and facilitators to handle and maneuver. Noodles bend. You can tie them in a knot. As a forgiving obstacle or a soft base of support, noodles are fun!

Noodle Balance

Learning Reinforced

Balance, body image, strength, cardiorespiratory fitness, endurance

Equipment

One noodle per child

Description

Ask the child to sit on a noodle the way he or she would sit on a swing. Assist with positioning as needed. Ask the child, "Can you sit so that you don't fall off?" If a child exhibits a lot of movement, ask, "Can you sit very still?" This will increase his or her ability to remain on the noodle.

Variations

Ask the child if he or she can sit without holding onto the noodle with his or her hands. Ask the child to kneel on a noodle. Ask the child if he or she can place it behind the back and under the armpits and recline. In each case, ask the child to hold the position, "Can you freeze or be a statue?" Gradually increase the length of time the child holds each position. To increase difficulty, while the child is holding the balanced position, move your hands in a back-and-forth motion behind him or her to add turbulence and challenge the balance.

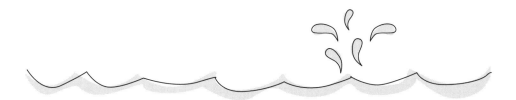

Noodle Structures

Learning Reinforced

Spatial orientation, submersion, concepts of in and out and over and under, color recognition

Equipment

A dozen or more pool noodles of different colors (Begin with primary colors—red, yellow, blue—and progress to secondary colors—purple, orange, and green. If available, use connector noodles, noodles with holes into which the ends of other noodles can be inserted.)

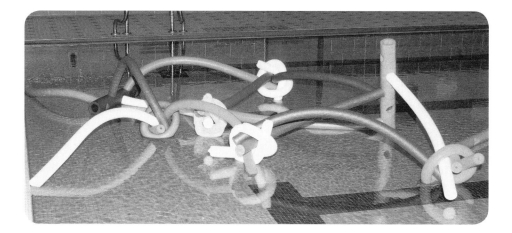

Description

Make a noodle structure. To anchor ends of noodles, tie one noodle in a knot and insert the end of another noodle into the knot (one knot can usually anchor three long noodles, each going out in a different direction) or use connector noodles. Bend the long noodles slightly to make arches above or on the water. Once you have made the structure, you can use it in a variety of ways.

- As an obstacle course—ask the child to enter the structure from one side, move through the structure by ducking under the "walls," and then move out the other end. Position the child on the opposite side of the structure from you and ask, "Can you come through the structure to me?" To make the task more difficult ask, "Can you come through without touching the noodles?"

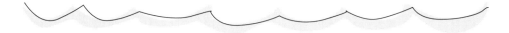

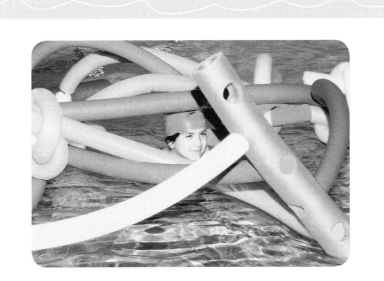

- As a house with doors of a variety of colors—ask the child to enter through one color and leave through another. Ask, "Can you come in through yellow?" When the child is inside, ask, "Can you go out through red?"
- As a group "popcorn" activity—gather the children around the outside of the structure. Ask them to move to the opposite side from wherever they are. If a child "pops" into a noodle room where another child already is, the first child in the room must "pop" to a different room.

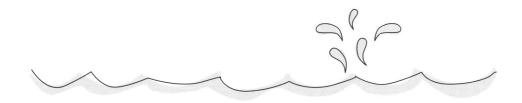

Higher and Higher, Lower and Lower

Learning Reinforced
Spatial orientation, directionality, submersion, breath control

Equipment
One noodle

Description
Using the side of the pool, ladder, or other fixed object as a brace, hold one end of the noodle in your hand and brace the other end.

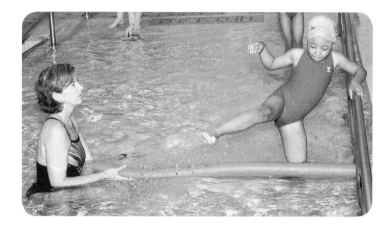

   Ask the child to go over or under the noodle. To go under, start with the noodle above water so that going under is easy. Gradually place the noodle lower and lower. To go over, start with the noodle on the bottom of the pool and gradually raise the noodle toward the surface. To keep the noodle submerged, sit or step on an end instead of holding it. Remind children submerging to hold their breath or blow bubbles.

Variations
Children will respond in a variety of ways to the request to go under the noodle. Each child engages differently, depending on a variety of factors including comfort with the task, flexibility, ability to submerge, height of the noodle, and general self-confidence. All responses can bring success and should be praised. Even the child who lifts the noodle to go under without submerging has successfully solved the problem. This is an advantage of the problem-solving approach. To increase difficulty, ask, "Can you go under without touching the noodle?" Change direction and increase difficulty by asking, "Can you go over backward?" Adding body-part orientation also adds challenge. Ask, "Can you go over with your left foot first?"

Noodle Balance Beam

Learning Reinforced
Balance, body image

Equipment
One noodle per child

Description
This activity requires three people. Begin in water chest high for the child. Two people stand on opposite ends of the noodle, anchoring it to the bottom of the pool. The noodle then becomes a balance beam for the child to walk on forward, backward, and sideward. Begin by asking the child, "Can you stand on the noodle?" Once the child can stand, ask him or her, "Can you walk on the noodle?" Praise any type of step the child takes, "Good walking!" or "Great step, you were balanced!" If the child has difficulty balancing in chest-high water, move to shoulder depth, but never deeper. The deeper water will provide greater support and aid balance. As the child becomes more confident, move to shallower water where more of the child's body is out of water and the setting is more like a balance beam on land.

Variations
Ask the child to walk with closed eyes. Ask the child to walk while keeping the arms crossed across his or her chest. Vary the type of step by asking the child if he or she can walk by alternating feet, walking with the left (or right) foot always first, or walking sideward.

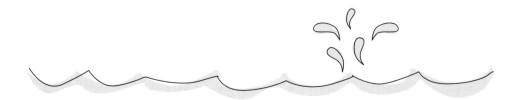

Noodle Locomotion

Learning Reinforced

Balance, strength, endurance, directionality, spatial orientation

Equipment

One noodle for each participant

Description

Ask the child, "Can you sit on your noodle like you are sitting on a swing?" Once the child is seated and balanced, present a variety of movement challenges, asking the child if he or she can move forward, backward, sideward, turn in circles, move to the left or right—all without falling off his or her noodle.

Variations

Specify parts of the body to be used, for example, "Can you move forward using just your arms? Can you move backward using just your legs? Can you move without using your arms or legs?" Add speed to the challenge by asking, "How fast can you move _____ using _____?" For additional variation, change the position of the noodle. Ask the child to sit straddling the noodle like riding a bicycle. Or challenge the child to place the noodle behind his or her back with the ends under his or her armpits and sit back like sitting in a recliner. Challenge the child in the recliner position to move forward feet first and to move backward. Increase the difficulty of any variation by challenging the child to travel a greater distance or travel faster. Add an obstacle course of floating objects to improve both motor control and spatial orientation.

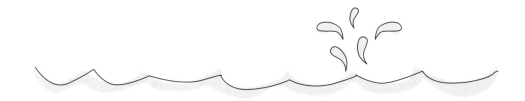

Parachutes*

A parachute is generally thought of as a piece of physical education equipment to be used on land. However, in the pool, a parachute can not only facilitate a variety of water learning activities but also be a catalyst for helping a child interact with larger groups of children. Most water learning activities are designed for individual children, partners, or small groups. A parachute is more suitable for large-group activities. For many parachute activities, group cooperation is needed for a successful outcome. The number of children available will determine the most appropriate size for the parachute. The larger the parachute, the more children needed for the activity to be successful. This expands water learning activities into birthday party and special-event programming.

Parachute Aerobics

Learning Reinforced
Grasp and squeeze, strength, endurance, cardiorespiratory fitness, laterality, directionality

Equipment
Parachute

Description
Spread the parachute open on the surface of the water. Ask the children to find places around the parachute and to grasp the edge of the chute. Facilitators may stand between children, also holding the parachute, or may stand behind a child, grasping the chute on top of the child's hands to facilitate grasp. When everyone is grasping the chute, ask the children, "Can we move our circle to the right?" Everyone should start moving to the right, holding tightly to the parachute. Then ask, "Can we move to the left?" As children become comfortable moving in each direction, add variations.

Variations
Ask the children, "Can we move faster? Can we move slower? Can we move very, very fast? Can we wiggle the parachute while we move?" Change the speed of the moving circle and the direction of travel to increase the effects of turbulence. The longer the circling continues, the more it challenges a child's cardiorespiratory system and develops strength and endurance. Sing a song while circling for additional respiratory enhancement.

---

*Sincere appreciation to adapted aquatics specialist Jean Skinner, Fairfax, Virginia, Parks and Recreation Department for her inspiring ideas on using parachutes in the pool.

Bouncy Chute

Learning Reinforced

Grasp and squeeze, hand and arm strength and endurance, balance

Equipment

Parachute, variety of medium and large lightweight balls

Description

Spread the parachute on top of the water, and ask the children to find places around the chute, grabbing its edge. Facilitators can intersperse themselves among the children, either next to a child or behind, helping the child grasp the chute. Place one or two balls onto the chute. Ask the children, "Can you make the balls bounce into the air?" Lifting the chute will also lift the balls. The higher the group lifts the chute, the higher the balls will go. A sharp lift of the chute will launch the balls into the air. Once the children figure out how to get the balls up, ask, "Can you make the balls go higher?"

Variations

Increase the number of balls on the chute. Then, ask the children, "Can we get all the balls into the air at the same time?" This requires everyone to work together as they bring the chute up and down. To further increase the difficulty, ask, "Can we move our chute to the right (circle right) while we pop the balls into the air?" Changing directions and lifting with shorter, quicker lifts will create "popcorn."

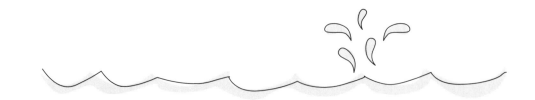

Oops!

Learning Reinforced

Grasp and squeeze, hand and arm strength and endurance, eye–hand coordination

Equipment

Parachute, variety of medium and large lightweight balls

Description

Begin the same as in Bouncy Chute. Once children learn how to bounce the balls into the air, ask, "Can you bounce the balls so that they fly off the chute?" This will require lifting one section while another section remains low. Challenge the children to try to bounce balls off the chute without allowing balls to bounce off the chute at their place. This requires additional timing for lifting and lowering the chute. If a ball leaves the chute, retrieve it, but wait to put it back until all the balls have been bounced off.

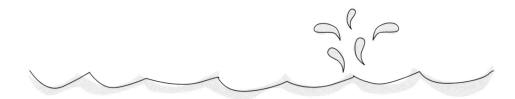

Switch

Learning Reinforced

Grasp and squeeze, hand and arm strength and endurance, spatial orientation, number recognition, memory

Equipment

Parachute

Description

Spread the parachute open on the surface of the water. Ask the children to find places around the parachute and to grasp the edge of the chute. Facilitators may stand between children and hold the parachute, or may stand behind a child, grasping the chute on top of the child's hands to facilitate grasp. When everyone is holding the chute, ask everyone participating to count off and remember his or her number. Ask the entire group to start lifting and lowering the parachute. Explain that when the chute goes up, you will call two numbers. The two people whose numbers you call must switch places by moving under the chute while it is in the air. Everyone on the edge must work to keep the chute up while the exchange takes place.

> ### Safety Tip
> The group should hold up the chute during the entire exchange. Watch to make sure no one gets caught under the chute as it comes down. On land this might not be a problem; however, in water, someone could get caught underwater.

Variation

Vary how many numbers you call. When you call more than two numbers, participants may move into any space that has been vacated.

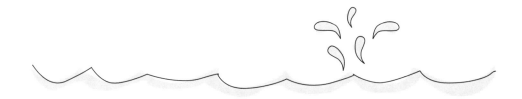

Chute Balance

Learning Reinforced
Grasp and squeeze, hand and arm strength and endurance, balance

Equipment
Parachute

Description
Spread the parachute open on the surface of the water. Ask the children to find places around the parachute and to grasp the edge of the chute. Facilitators may stand between children and hold the parachute, or they may stand behind a child, grasping the chute on top of the child's hands to facilitate grasp. When everyone is holding the chute, ask everyone if they can lean back slightly, making the chute taut. Then ask the children, "Who thinks they can make a statue on the parachute?" Select a brave volunteer to try. He or she should climb onto the parachute and take a place in the middle. Once in place, he or she assumes a sitting or kneeling position (hands and knees or just knees), creating a very still statue. The parachute will still have enough give to make balance difficult. Remind holders to lean back to keep the chute tight.

Variations
Count how long a child can hold his or her statue. Ask a second child to imitate the statue the first child makes. Provide creative stimulation for statues. Ask, "Can you be a puppy?" or "Can you be a chair?"

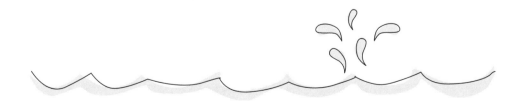

Free Ride

Learning Reinforced

Grasp and squeeze, hand and arm strength and endurance, balance

Equipment

Parachute

Description

Spread the parachute open on the surface of the water. Ask the children to find places around the parachute and to grasp the edge of the chute. Facilitators may stand between children and hold the parachute, or they may stand behind a child, grasping the chute on top of the child's hands to facilitate grasp. When everyone is holding the chute, ask everyone if they can lean back slightly, making the chute taut. Ask the children, "Who would like a ride on the parachute?" Select a brave volunteer to ride. He or she then climbs onto the parachute and takes a place in the middle. The riding child can sit or recline. Once settled, ask, "Can we move the parachute around to the right and take _____ for a ride?" The entire group circles slowly to the right while the volunteer rides the parachute. It is important to pull back slightly and hold tightly to the chute because the riding child will add weight.

Variations

Increase the speed of the ride. Jiggle the chute to provide a bumpy ride or to simulate a bucking bronco, vibrating rocket ship, or Quidditch broom (depending on the age of the children). Yes, adults can ride too, further stimulating the children to "make that chute really move!"

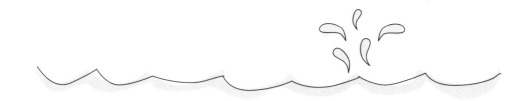

Poly Shapes

Poly shapes are exceedingly user friendly for water learning. Produced by Poly Enterprises (www.polyenterprises.com), Monrovia, California, poly objects sink to the bottom of the pool; stay in place even on a slope; come in a variety of colors, shapes, sizes, and purposes; and dry easily for storage. Examples of poly shapes include the following:

alphabet letters	numbers
arrows	puzzles
footprints (side specific)	shark and frog shapes
geometric shapes	spots
handprints (side specific)	stars

Uses of poly shapes in water learning are limited only by creativity. Following are just a few examples.

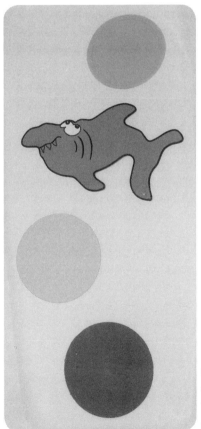

Photo by Sue Grosse

Alphabet Spots

Learning Reinforced

Letter recognition, math, number recognition, spelling, visual perception

Equipment

Two sets of poly alphabets and numbers

Description

Scatter the poly letters and numbers. Ask the children to stand on specific letters or numbers as you name them. Increase the difficulty by asking the children to step on their initials, letters in their name or easy words, the numbers in their age or address, and so on. To work on spelling, ask the children to step out the

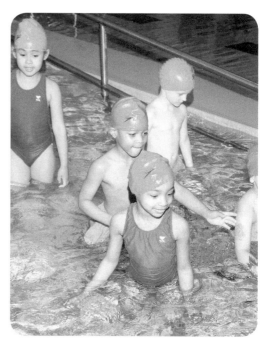

spelling. Children may put their face in the water to look at the letters. Cue them, "Don't forget to hold your breath and blow bubbles."

Variations

Increase feedback by asking the child to say the letter before stepping on it. Ask the child to name each letter as he or she spells a word and then say the word when spelling is completed. Ask the child to verbalize a math problem as he or she steps it out.

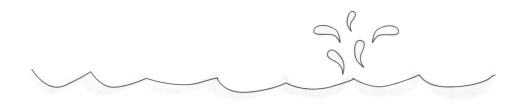

Safe Spot

Learning Reinforced
Auditory perception, safety skills, following directions

Equipment
One poly spot for each child

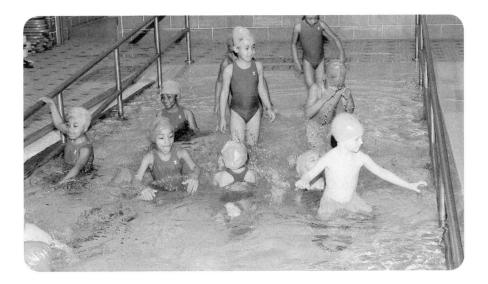

Description
Use the poly spot as a sit-upon. Ask children to remain seated on their spot until receiving permission to enter the water or, if in water, until beginning an activity. You can also designate the spot as the location a child should return to after completing a challenge or job.

Variation
If a child needs additional cuing to find his or her spot, ask the child to select a spot that matches his or her swim attire, swim cap, or colored wristband.

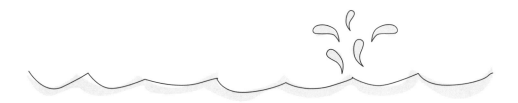

Be a Star

Learning Reinforced

Auditory perception, creativity, balance, spatial orientation

Equipment

A dozen large poly stars or spots in various colors, music

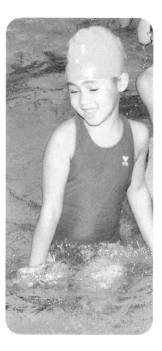

Description

Scatter the stars on the bottom of the pool. Ask the child, "Can you move around without stepping on any of the stars?" Once the child demonstrates that he or she can accomplish this, ask, "Can you move around without stepping on any stars until you hear music? When you hear music, can you stand on a star and perform for me? You can do anything you want that goes with the music." Praise all performances. Stop and start the music several times. Keep the intervals between changes no longer than 15 seconds.

Variations

Change the type of music. Start with music familiar to the child. Gradually add music with different characteristics to encourage different movements.

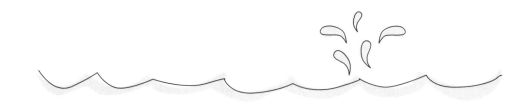

Musical Spots

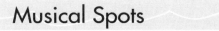

Learning Reinforced

Auditory perception, motor control

Equipment

Six to eight poly spots (if working with a group, at least one spot for each person), music

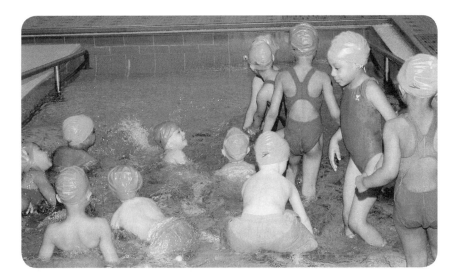

Description

Place spots on the bottom of the pool in a random pattern, allowing space to move around between spots. Ask the children if they can move around the pool space without stepping on or touching any of the spots. Play music while they are moving. Then ask, "When the music stops, can you find a spot and stand on it (or sit, kneel, or make a statue)?" When the music starts again, ask the children to continue moving.

Variations

Increase the difficulty by asking the children if they can stop on a spot of a different color each time the music stops. Gradually reduce verbal cues until children are responding only to whether the music is playing or not. Vary the size of the spots. Smaller spots are harder to target and stand on without moving. Reverse the process by asking the children if they can walk and step on the spots and jump off when the music stops.

On the Spot

Learning Reinforced
Balance, body image

Equipment
One poly spot per person

Description
Begin in water that is chest deep for the child. Ask the child, "Can you stand with both feet on the spot and hold this position for five seconds like a statue?" If the child can accomplish this task, progressively add these positions to the challenge:

- Stand with eyes closed (which may be combined with any of the following poses).
- Stand with arms crossed across the chest (which may be combined with any of the following poses).
- Stand on one foot.
- Stand on one foot, with the bottom of the other foot placed against the knee.
- Move the arms from a position at the sides to fully extended overhead.
- Perform a variety of Simon Says activities while on the spot.
- Play Follow the Leader, with each participant on his or her own spot, imitating the arm actions of the leader.

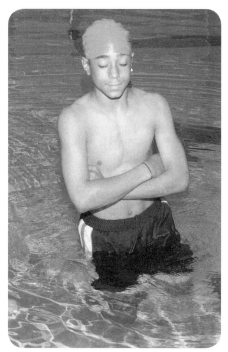

Variations
Gradually move to shallower water. The shallower the water, the more difficult the balance challenge will be and the more closely the challenge will approximate balance skills on land. As a child performs any of the On the Spot challenges, stand behind the child and move your hands and arms back and forth underwater to increase turbulence. It is more difficult to maintain balance in turbulent water than in still water.

Poly Trail

Learning Reinforced

Balance, laterality, direction-ality, spatial orientation, gait training

Equipment

Poly footprints, arrows, frogs, and sharks

Description

Arrange a footprint trail on the bottom of the pool. Begin with an easy trail: short steps alternating left and right. Ask the child, "Can you walk our trail, placing your feet on our poly footprints?" Encourage the child to match left and right feet to the footprints, even if that means changing step length.

Variations

As the child accomplishes this task, adjust the trail to vary the size of the steps, direction of travel, and foot pattern. Add obstacles such as sharks or frogs to step over. Increase the challenge by asking the child if he or she can move along the trail without using the arms for balance (the child can place his or her arms across the chest or on top of the head). Increase cardiorespiratory fitness by asking the child if he or she can move faster and jog or run the trail. Set the trails in a variety of patterns to encourage continuous movement and aerobic activity. Additional variations include the following:

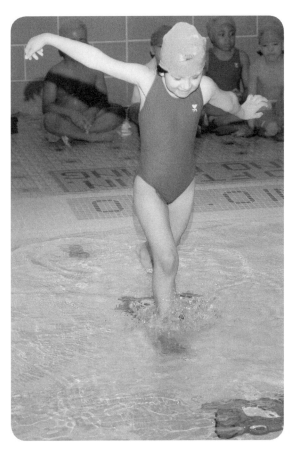

- Easy steps and steps over obstacles such as frogs and sharks
- Jumps and jumps over frogs and sharks
- Heel-toe steps with crossover steps where one foot must step across the midline of the body (crossing the other foot)
- Mixed problems
- Changes of direction and following arrows

Spot Tag

Learning Reinforced

Spatial orientation, counting

Equipment

One poly spot for each child

Description

Scatter the spots. Ask the children if they know how to play tag, and then explain the rules of Spot Tag. One person is It. The other children move around the area while the child who is It tries to tag them. Children cannot be tagged if they are standing on a spot. However, they may only stay on a spot for three seconds and must count the seconds out loud. If tagged, that child becomes It and cannot tag back his or her tagger.

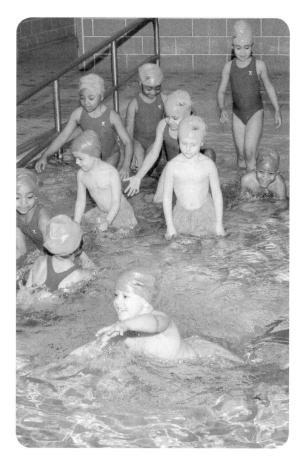

Variations

Increase the distance between the spots, making it more difficult to stay on a spot all the time. Reduce the number of safe spots by making only spots of a certain color safe.

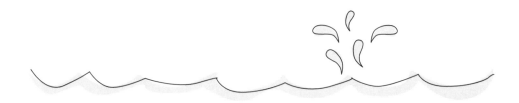

Steps

Aqua steps, such as those used in aquatic step aerobics, available from Speedo (www.speedo.com), Los Angeles, California, can provide a variety of water learning experiences. Step activities, such as traditional step aerobics, gait training, and an obstacle trail, can improve balance, laterality, and directionality; increase cardiorespiratory function, strength, and endurance; and challenge a child's ability to imitate and follow directions.

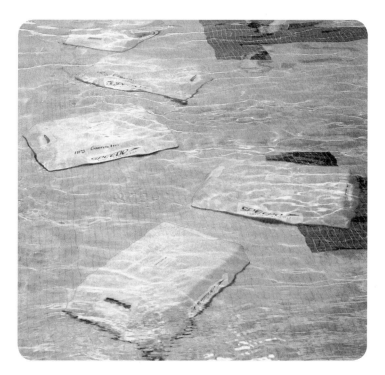

Statue

Learning Reinforced

Balance, imitation, following directions, creativity

Equipment

One aqua step for each child

Description

Ask the child, "Can you stand on your step and stay still like a statue?" When the child accomplishes this, ask for different kinds of statues, including objects, animals, activities, and feelings and fantasy (e.g., an angry statue or a monster statue). Between statue challenges allow a "melt" period, when the child can collapse and shake out limbs.

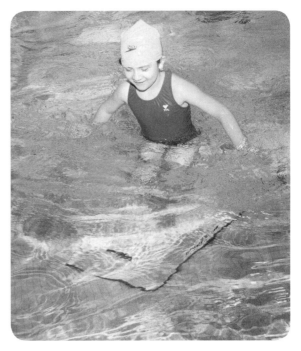

Variations

If working with a group, ask one child to be leader, or statue maker, who strikes a pose. Ask the other children to assume the same pose as the statue maker. If working with one child, ask the child to let you "sculpt" him or her. The child stands like a statue while you, as the sculptor, move the statue into different positions. Ask the child, "Can you hold the shape I sculpt?" Praise the child as he holds each position steady. Gradually increase the time the child holds a position before moving on to the next.

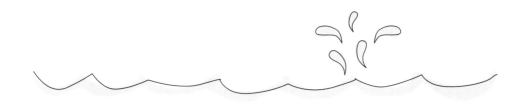

Step Trail

Learning Reinforced

Balance, laterality, directionality, gait training

Equipment

Five to seven aqua steps

Description

Create a trail by placing the steps with narrow ends facing each other. Initially, the steps should be in a straight line with the steps almost touching each other. Ask the child, "Can you walk from one step to the next without touching the bottom of the pool?"

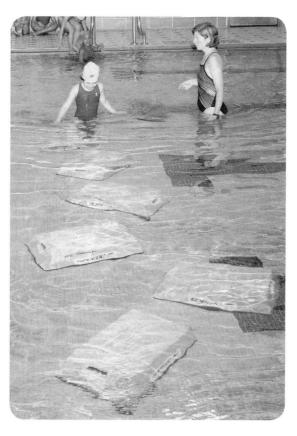

Variations

As participants become confident, increase the distance between steps. As proficiency increases, place steps at angles to each other to vary direction. Ask the child to walk backward or sideward. Ask several children to move on the trail at the same time from opposite ends. This adds the challenge of passing each other while maintaining balance and not touching. Not touching teaches children to respect each other's space as well as use their arms appropriately for balance.

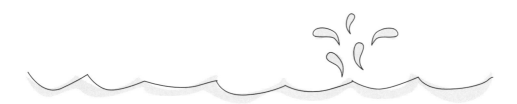

Step Aerobics

Learning Reinforced

Cardiorespiratory fitness, endurance, strength, gait training

Equipment

One aqua step for each child

Description

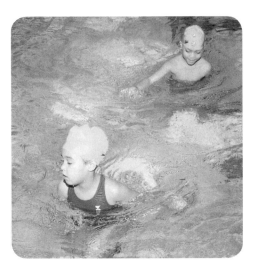

Yes, children can do aqua step aerobics. Stepping, hopping, and jumping on and off an aqua step to lively music can build fitness and help develop longer time-on-task behavior. Start without music. Ask the child, "Can you step onto the step?" Offer the child your hand to assist with balance if the child appears reluctant. Once the child has stepped onto the platform, ask, "Can you step off?" At this point, the child may step off in any direction. Once the child has mastered stepping onto and off of the step, add more specific stepping patterns.

- Step on and step off forward, walk around the step, and repeat.
- Step on and step off forward, turn around, and repeat facing the opposite direction.
- Step on and step off backward, and repeat.
- Step on, step to the side, and step off sideward. Repeat to the opposite side for step off.
- Step on, turn around, and step off forward. Turn around and repeat.
- Step on, turn around, step off backward, and repeat.
- Step on, perform an arm exercise or wave, and step off (as desired).

Variations

Encourage the child to make the stepping continuous. Add music with a strong beat. Ask the child, "Can you step to the beat?" If the child has difficulty hearing the beat of the music, clap the beat first, asking the child to clap with you. When the child can clap the beat, add stepping. Playing Follow the Leader as a group activity enhances creativity because children strive to outperform each other. Pace determines the cardiorespiratory benefit. Music with a slower tempo makes stepping easier. Picking up the pace increases the demand on a child not only for motor processing but also for cardiorespiratory fitness.

Washcloths

The washcloth is a wonderful piece of water learning equipment. Easy to obtain, uncomplicated to use, and easy for a child to grasp in his or her hand, the washcloth takes the shape of the objects on which it is placed. Washcloths are colorful, squishy, familiar from home, and each child can have his or her own. Because washcloths are used in activities of daily living, there is great potential for carryover into personal hygiene skills and academic reinforcement.

Washcloth Fitness

Learning Reinforced
Strength, endurance, cardiorespiratory fitness, body image, kinesthetic awareness

Equipment
One washcloth per child, aqua steps or poly shapes

Description
Asking the child to carry a washcloth in his or her hand enhances any arm activity, whether it is a specific exercise or just using arms for balance while moving through the water. The wet cloth adds weight, which you can adjust to the size, grip strength, and abilities of the child. The smaller the cloth, the lighter the weight. And that weight increases the child's awareness of where the hand and arm are in space. Ask the child to perform water learning activities using aqua steps or poly shapes while carrying a washcloth.

Variations
A loose cloth, held by one corner, has drag. It will pull back on the hand and arm. A cloth folded or wadded into the hand will have a more concentrated weight. This means the cloth can accommodate the grasp characteristics of the child. Alternate dragging and holding the cloth for increased variety. Initially, the child should keep the cloths underwater where they weigh less. Add action just above the surface as strength improves.

Wash Me

Learning Reinforced

Body image, daily living activities, safety (shower first), kinesthetic awareness, washing

Equipment

One washcloth per child

Description

Although the real washing should happen in the shower before entering the pool, using a washcloth in the pool to wash body parts is a fun activity to start children on the road to independent self-cleanliness. Ask the child to name his or her body parts as he or she washes them with pool water. If a child is hesitant to enter the pool, washing can take place on a zero-depth ramp or on stairs.

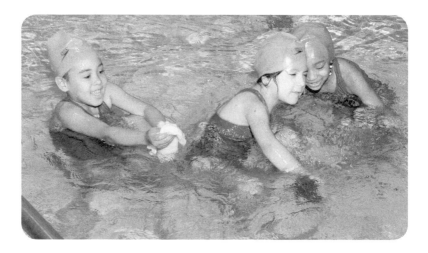

A child can also wash while sitting on a poly spot on the pool deck. A child can get his or her cloth as wet—or keep it as dry—as he or she wants. If an adult washes a child, using just a bit more pressure than usual can provide kinesthetic feedback for identification of body parts and aid in differentiating one part from another. Washcloths come in a variety of textures and fabric weights. Using fabric besides what is typically used for washcloths provides greater texture variety. Encourage the child's physical and verbal participation. Having the child repeat, "Now I'm washing my _____," reinforces body-part identification and task accomplishment.

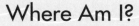

Where Am I?

Learning Reinforced

Laterality, directionality, spatial orientation, body image, grasp and release

Equipment

One washcloth per child

Description

This activity is all about where the child's body is in relation to the washcloth. Initiate the activity by asking, "Can you put the washcloth _____?" or "Can you put yourself _____?" or

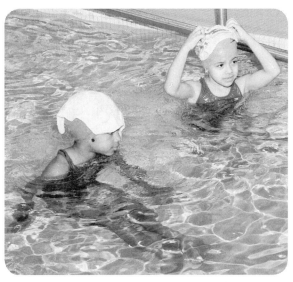

similar questions related to cloth or body placement. A variety of positions for the cloth and child will result. Here are some examples:

Can you put the washcloth on top of you?

Can you put the washcloth under you?

Can you put the washcloth on your foot?

Can you put the washcloth behind your back?

Can you go under the washcloth?

Can you stand on top of the washcloth?

Can you stand to the right of your washcloth?

Start with very simple relationships and gradually progress to more complicated ones. If a child places the cloth correctly, repeat the arrangement with praise and an affirming statement, "Great job, you have the washcloth behind your back." If the child places the washcloth incorrectly, ask the child questions to help clarify inaccurate body parts and locations, such as, "Is that really your _____ or is it your _____? Is that over or under?" Try to cue the child to correct his or her own errors. As a last resort, correctly describe the position the child is in and go on to another challenge. Later, return to the challenge that proved difficult.

Variation

Perform this activity with a Wonderboard (described in the next section) or a poly spot.

Wonderboards*

Wider and more concave than a standard kickboard, a Wonderboard is made from high-density foam. Although a regular foam kickboard would be feasible for the activities presented here, Wonderboards provide a more stable base of support for both balance activities and aerobics.

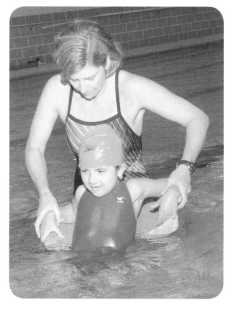

Balance Board

Learning Reinforced
Balance, body image

Equipment
One Wonderboard per child

Description
Hold the Wonderboard behind the child with hands on the narrow sides, and ask the child, "Can you sit on the Wonderboard?" Submerge the board to just below the child's buttocks, holding it steady while the child sits.

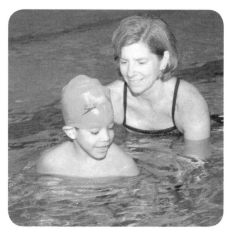

Continue to hold the board steady as the child adjusts his or her weight until balanced. Gradually decrease the amount of stabilization you provide, allowing the board to move with the action of the water. Encourage the child to stay on the board, using his or her arms underwater for balance. Count the number of seconds the child can sit before he or she tips off.

---

*Wonderboards, available from Aquatics by Sprint (www.sprintaquatics.com), San Luis Obispo, California, are specially designed kickboards.

Variations

Once a child has mastered a comfortable seated balance, encourage the child to get onto the board without assistance. To increase the difficulty of sitting on the board, move your hands back and forth behind the board underwater to create turbulence. The task will also be more difficult if you ask the child to close his or her eyes.

Safety Tip

Initially, balancing may be difficult. Stay close by to help the child right himself or herself should a fall occur. Some children will be comfortable regaining their footing. Others will be in a potential drowning situation and will need assistance in regaining a standing position.

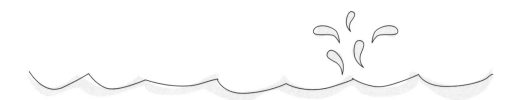

Tippy Board

Learning Reinforced

Balance, body image, spatial orientation, safety (recovering from fall)

Equipment

One Wonderboard per child

Description

Once a child masters independent seated balance, it is important for the child to learn how to fall off his or her board and recover to a safe standing or breathing position. Wonderboards are great fun. However, many of the more vigorous activities may involve falling off. Teaching recovery is an important safety precaution. Begin by discussing briefly what could happen if the child falls off. Accept what the child proposes. Then ask the child to purposely tip over by leaning gently to one side. As the child falls, let his or her body completely leave the board and float free in the water. Then provide a gentle underarm assist to stand or assist to back float, which is a safe resting position.

Variations

Once the child can gently ease off, ask the child to pretend he or she is an object that has more force—a monster truck, rocket, train, plane, and so on—objects that will leave the board more quickly, more unexpectedly, or with greater impact, causing further submersion. Pretending the board is a bucking bronco or mountain bike in rough terrain also provides good analogies.

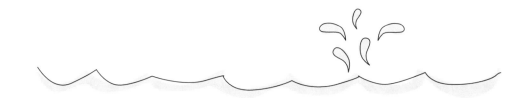

Advanced Balance Board

Learning Reinforced
Balance, body image

Equipment
One Wonderboard per child, a variety of objects to throw and catch

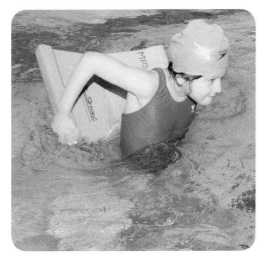

Description
Once the child masters independent seated balance and can comfortably fall off the board and recover, you can add greater challenges.

Can you kneel on the board?

Can you stand on the board?

Can you sit on the board and tuck your hands under your bottom?

Can you sit on the board and toss and catch a ball?

Can you sit on the board and play catch with me?

Variation
Ask the child to perform the balance activities while wearing a blindfold.

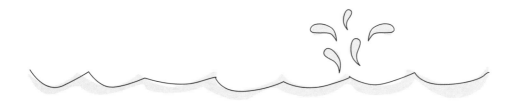

Wonderboard Aerobics

Learning Reinforced
Cardiorespiratory fitness, strength, endurance, balance, body image

Equipment
One Wonderboard per child, music (optional)

Description
Encourage children seated on boards to try a variety of locomotor activities. If they fall off, they should just get back on again. Adjust the speed of performance to develop strength. Adjust the length of the activity to develop endurance. Vary the motor activity without stopping the general flow of action. One pattern should flow into the next. The following are examples of ways to finish the question "Can you use your arms to _____?"

- Move forward, backward, and sideward
- Spin in circles
- Look like a paddling dog, like a fish tail, like you are continually opening curtains
- Pull
- Push
- Bounce

Or use these examples to finish the question "Using your legs for locomotion and keeping your arms crossed over your chest or your hands on your shoulders, can you _____?"

- Move forward, backward, or sideward
- Spin in circles
- Kick like you're kicking a ball, kick like you're riding a bicycle, or kick like you're jogging
- Move back first, move belly first, move knees first, or move shoulders first

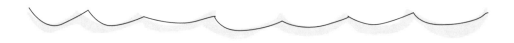

Ask the child to try to use the board in a reclining position. Place the board behind the child, lengthwise behind the spine, with the lower edge of the board at hip level. Hold the bottom corners with each hand and let the child recline back onto the board. Ask the child to use just the legs for locomotion while trying the challenges for legs just described. It will be especially challenging for the child to use the bottoms of his or her feet to pull water, moving the body toward the feet.

Variations

In any position, vary the speed of travel, direction, and quality of movement (gentle, forceful, tiny, large, angry, scary, happy, bouncy, soft). Ask children to form pairs. The partners should either hook elbows, or you could designate a touch point (backs remaining touching, for example). From this position, partners must accomplish the movement tasks described earlier. Either alone or with a partner, the children perform a variety of relay races. Either alone or with a partner, the children perform the movement exploration activities described in that section.

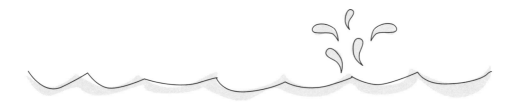

Wonderboard Spud

Learning Reinforced
Balance, eye–hand coordination, throwing and catching

Equipment
One Wonderboard per child, a soft ball

Description
Spud is a group activity. The children gather in a circle on their boards. One person is It. That person tosses the ball into the air inside the circle and calls the name of another child. The child whose name is called must get the ball, either catching it or fetching it. Everyone else moves away from the child called. When the child has the ball he or she calls "Stop." The child with the ball tosses the ball and tries to hit another child. Shots to the head are not allowed. If he or she hits a child, that child is It and gets a letter: S, P, U, D, in that order. If the toss does not hit another player, the thrower gets a letter. The players re-form the circle, and the cycle begins again. The first person to get SPUD loses and the game starts over from the beginning. All players must remain on their boards the entire time. If someone falls off, he or she must remount the board before moving to avoid getting hit or to toss. Players off their boards are fair game. This is not an elimination game.

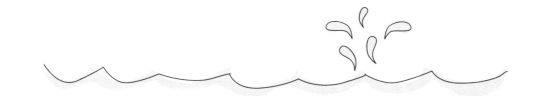

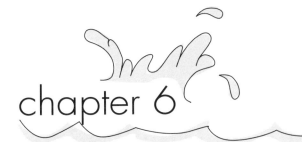

chapter 6

Planning and Assessment

Selecting activities for a water learning lesson depends on a variety of factors, including equipment available, physical setting, and time frame. However, the learning needs of the child should be your primary concern. When choosing activities, select those that reinforce the learning taking place outside the water environment.

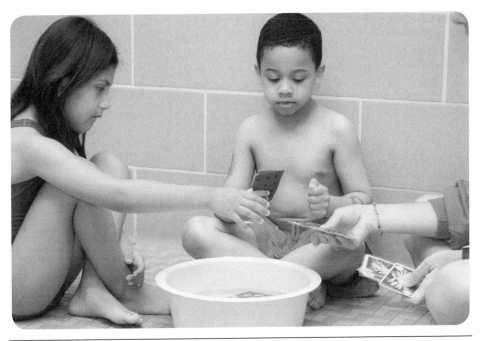

Select water activities that reinforce the learning that takes place outside the water environment.

Planning for Water Learning Integration

To coordinate water learning with academic and therapeutic goals, use the Water Learning Planning Chart (see table 6.1). Across the top of the chart are specific learning activity areas. The left side lists areas of growth and development. To complete the chart, find out what is being done in each activity area (top row) to improve each area of development (left column).

Find out what learning objectives are planned in the child's academic and physical education classes and whether the child is receiving therapy. Use that information to fill in the blank spaces in the classroom, physical education, and therapeutic interventions columns on the chart (see table 6.2). Use the categories in the left-hand column to clarify specific information. Add information categories to the left column if the child has learning goals that do not fit existing groups.

Table 6.1 Water Learning Planning Chart

	Classroom	Physical education	Therapeutic interventions	Water learning
Academics				
Motor development				
Physical fitness				
Social development				
Behavior				
Self-esteem				
Activities of daily living				

Table 6.2 Sample Water Learning Planning Chart

Sally's water learning planning chart	Classroom (Sally is in an age 4-5 pre-school.)	Physical education (Sally is in a preschool play group.)	Therapeutic interventions (Sally sees a therapist to help overcome attention-deficit/ hyperactivity disorder.)	Water learning
Academics	Word recognition of common objects, addition	Words that match motor skills	Card matching game during play therapy	
Motor development	Holding a pencil correctly for printing	Throwing a bean-bag at a target	Drawing during play therapy	
Physical fitness	Hand strength for writing	Hand/arm strength for throwing	Game of catch	
Social development	Sharing with one other person	Playing a target game with another person	Appropriate on-task interaction with the therapist	
Behavior	Staying on task for longer than 5 minutes	Staying on the same task the group is on	Staying on task with the therapist	
Self-esteem	Successful academic activities	Successful activities with the group	Successful activities in therapy, reduction in random movement around the therapy room	
Activities of daily living	Sally does fine in this area.	Sally does fine and can tie her own tennis shoes.	Sally puts on her own jacket at the end of the session.	

Once you have entered the information, note the learning needs of the child based on the information in the chart. For example, Sally needs activities based on developing the following skills:

- Letter and word recognition
- Hand and arm strength
- Targeting
- Sharing with one or two other children
- Exhibiting on-task behavior

Sally's facilitator goes to the section of the activity finder that lists learning and motor development concepts (pages v to xiii) and selects water learning activities appropriate for Sally's learning needs. Those activities are entered on the Water Learning Planning Chart, right column. Because Sally will participate in water learning in her therapy setting and at home, the activities in chapter 4 are the most appropriate. Sally's facilitator chooses Picture Identification, Wring Out, Squeeze, and Fill the Bucket. The facilitator enters these activities onto Sally's Water Learning Planning Chart (see table 6.3).

Once you have completed a water learning chart for your child, you must organize the selected activities into a water learning session. These guidelines will help you organize an effective water learning session:

- Plan only as many activities as can be directly supervised by adults.
- After the child tries the initial task, give him or her freedom to experiment.
- Plan for progression, start with activities in which the child gets only a little wet, and gradually work up to a final activity in which the entire body is in contact with the water. A child who gets totally wet at the start of a lesson may end up chilled by the time the lesson is over. Children who are hesitant about the water experience may need to work up to getting really wet.
- Work from easy to difficult tasks, old to new, familiar to unfamiliar, large motor to small motor, short sequences to longer sequences.
- Select activities that use a variety of muscle groups and motor skills.
- After the initial lesson, include a combination of new and repeated activities in each session.
- At the conclusion of each lesson, allow time for creative exploration using equipment from that day's activity. Ask questions like, "What else can you do with _____?" or "Show me _____ another way?"
- Involve the child in the cleanup process. Children can help empty and dry equipment and should be working on drying and dressing themselves.

Table 6.3　Sample Completed Water Learning Planning Chart

Sally's water learning planning chart	Classroom (Sally is in an age 4-5 pre-school.)	Physical education (Sally is in a preschool play group.)	Therapeutic interventions (Sally sees a therapist to help overcome attention-deficit/ hyperactivity disorder.)	Water learning
Academics	Word recognition of common objects, addition	Words that match motor skills	Card matching game during play therapy	Picture Identification
Motor development	Holding a pencil correctly for printing	Throwing a beanbag at a target	Drawing during play therapy	Wring Out
Physical fitness	Hand strength for writing	Hand/arm strength for throwing	Game of catch	Squeeze
Social development	Sharing with one other person	Playing a target game with another person	Appropriate on-task interaction with the therapist	Fill the Bucket (large bucket, work with partner)
Behavior	Staying on task for longer than 5 minutes	Staying on the same task the group is on	Staying on task with the therapist	Fill the Bucket
Self-esteem	Successful academic activities	Successful activities with the group	Successful activities in therapy, reduction in random movement around the therapy room	Squeeze (aim at target)
Activities of daily living	Sally does fine in this area.	Sally does fine and can tie her own tennis shoes.	Sally puts on her own jacket at the end of the session.	Wring Out (washcloth)

- Whatever the lesson, be sure to allow enough time. Most water learning sessions take about half a day, especially those that require changing clothes. It is better to plan too few activities and have time left over than to try to do too much and run out of time, particularly if a shortage of time means you have to do tasks for the child, such as cleanup and dressing, that he or she could be learning to do for himself or herself. If you have too much time, sit down afterward and talk about the activities with the child.

Once planning is complete, carry out your plan. Then after the activity, make notes to record general information and to serve as helpful hints for future activities. To keep a more specific record of a child's participation and progress in water learning activities, add specific assessment documentation.

Assessing Water Learning

Assessment is an important part of any water learning program. Because physical activity in the water must be integrated with land-based academic activities and therapeutic goals, knowledge of the child's participation and progress is important. Perceptual-motor development is an integral component of learning style. Physical fitness plays a key role in development of motor skills. Control of large-muscle groups directly affects the fine motor control needed for writing and other manual-dexterity tasks. These are only a few of the myriad interactions taking place daily in the growth and development of every child. Gaining information about strengths and weaknesses in one area often provides clues to developmental needs in other areas.

Assessment provides information about these interactions, pinpointing those needing remediation and highlighting those that can be used to facilitate successful activity engagement. This is particularly important for children who have reached the age of formal education, whether preschool or kindergarten. You assess in order to plan future activities and document current success.

More specific reasons for assessment include the following:

- Program entry—to determine the current level of function before entry into a formal educational program
- Planning—to set individualized goals and objectives for participation in any program, class, or therapeutic treatment
- Documentation of progress—to compare current function with program entry or past level of function
- Confirmation of opinion—to lend support to observations and opinions regarding a child's development, needs, and progress

- Facilitation of team collaboration—to provide information for other professionals working with the child, thus facilitating coordination of programming
- Easing program transfer—to foster inclusion in regular aquatic and education programs by preparing a child to meet future assessment expectations

An assessment should yield information regarding a variety of areas of growth and development. These include the following:

- **Communication** refers to how a child receives and sends information to and from other people. Assessment of communication involves determining both expressive and receptive capabilities. Assessment of communication also includes determining if there is a preference for or deficit in auditory, visual, tactile, and kinesthetic communication forms.
- **Cognition** refers to how well a child understands information communicated through the various communication formats. Cognition also involves processing that information and the ability to express the results of that processing. Cognition is how a child accumulates information, and it can reflect intellectual level.

- **Motor development** includes, but is not limited to, motor patterns, reflexes, motor planning, and motor skills.
- **Physical fitness** consists of five components: strength, endurance, cardiorespiratory fitness, flexibility, and body composition.
- **Social and emotional development** includes arousal level, temperament, interaction with others, and play stage of development (singular, parallel, or interactive).

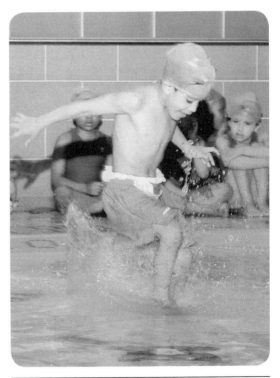

Perceptual-motor factors affect all areas of child growth and development.

Water activities are great for increasing cardio-respiratory fitness.

Each of the areas of perceptual-motor development deserves attention during the assessment process. These include the following:

- **Body image**—how well a child can identify and control all major body parts
- **Balance**—how much motor control a child has when moving in ways that challenge gravity
- **Laterality**—how well a child can differentiate the right and left sides of the body and perform tasks that require crossing the midline of the body
- **Directionality**—how well a child can move up, down, backward, forward, sideward, diagonally, and in combinations of all directions
- **Spatial orientation**—how well a child can move in relation to other objects and people, making appropriate movement choices with motor control
- **Ocular pursuit**—how well a child can visually track moving objects and plan motor activities in relation to these objects

Pool Activity Learning Chart

Table 6.4, Pool Activity Learning Chart, contains abbreviated activity descriptions that correspond to the water learning activities described in chapter 5. The purpose of each activity is to orient the child to other pursuits. The chart also lists the skills you can assess as the child participates.

The Pool Activity Learning Chart is a detailed reference document to help you plan and assess over time so that you can note and track a child's progress. No matter who provides the water learning experience—a classroom teacher, therapist, recreation professional, aquatic specialist, or parent—using the information obtained through this type of assessment and planning will make it easier to integrate water learning with information from all disciplines. And that is the ultimate goal of water learning, a coordinated reinforcement and support of all aspects of a child's education through activities in water.

Use the Pool Activity Learning Chart to determine which activities to use for specific assessment purposes. For example, if your child particularly enjoys working with noodles, which assessments can you integrate into the noodle activity sessions? Find noodles in the left column. Then read across to determine the developmental areas that noodle activities can assess (laterality, directionality, spatial orientation, balance, arm and leg strength and endurance, endurance). Or, if you want to assess balance and gait, for example, read down the right column to locate all the activity categories that can assess balance and gait (enhanced movement exploration, poly shapes, steps, Wonderboards, big boat, noodles, parachutes).

Table 6.4   Pool Activity Learning Chart

Category	Activity	Purpose
Big boat	Match colors by sorting into color bags Climb over Balance	Orientation to • Water • Space • Object manipulation Assesses • Color recognition • Matching • Balance • Strength • Flexibility • Muscle tone
Basic movement exploration	Establish the space Move around the space • Faster and slower • Backward and forward • Turn while moving Move without touching • People • Floating obstacles • Obstacles that are placed or thrown	Orientation to • Water • Space • Information source Assesses • Listening • Direction following • Problem solving • Preferred movement • Extraneous movement • Muscle tone • Endurance • Spatial orientation • Motor control
Enhanced movement exploration	Move around space • Size of movement (big steps, bigger, giant, small, smaller, tiny, showing toes, showing heels) • Height of movement (close to ceiling, close to bottom) • Animals (elephant, lion, dog, fish) • Moving vehicles (car, rocket, train) Move with sound • Animal and machine • Loud, louder, very loud, soft, whisper Move with purpose • Completing a task • Performing a job	Orientation to • Splash • Waves • Submersion Assesses • Range of motion • Balance • Endurance • Respiratory capacity • Cardiovascular fitness • Elementary experiences

(continued)

Table 6.4 *(continued)*

Category	Activity	Purpose
Clothing	Wear in water (locomotion and swim) Disrobe Re-dress	Orientation to • Added weight and resistance Assesses • Strength • Skill in daily living activities
Cone academics	Match number count, perform math processes, and match objects and functions	Orientation to • Submersion • Object retrieval Assesses • Matching • Number and letter recognition • Object and function relationships • Grasp and release • Breath holding
Interpretive movement	Lion Hunt (specific tasks will vary based on goals set into the story) • Put on pack, pick up spear, put on hat • Start hiking • Uphill and downhill • Cross muddy stream • Hear something in bushes • Hide • Climb tree and swing on branch • Climb down • Run back to camp Listen and move according to fantasy Listen and move to nonsense words	Orientation to • Following demonstration • Locomotion through water Assesses • Range of motion • Ability to copy • Endurance • Other skills, based on story • Imagination
Jobs	Listen to the job being presented Perform the job • Match • Retrieve • Sort Return to the start	Orientation to • Submersion • Breath control Assesses • Skills required by assignment • Task completion • Direction following related to start, type of job, and completion

Category	Activity	Purpose
Noodles	Climb over noodle Move under noodle Balance on noodle Move through structure Move while balancing on noodle	Orientation to • Submersion Assesses • Laterality • Directionality • Spatial orientation • Balance • Arm and leg strength and endurance • Endurance
Parachutes	Grasp and hold chute Lift and lower chute Walk or jog while holding chute Shake chute Balance on chute Ride on chute	Orientation to • Group activity Assesses • Grasp • Hand and arm strength and endurance • Endurance • Balance
Poly shapes	Balance • 2 feet • 1 foot • 1 foot, arms crossed • 1 foot, arms crossed, foot on knee • Eyes closed • With waves Traverse the trail • Alternating feet • Crossover steps • Hop • Jump Following trail directions • Arrows • Lines • Signs Traverse trail obstacles • Frogs and sharks • Steps	Orientation to • Locomotion through water Assesses • Balance • Gait • Mobility • Direction following • Spatial orientation
Steps	Follow a trail, stepping from step to step Step on and off Step on and off with direction change Step on and off in tempo	Orientation to • Locomotion in water Assesses • Gait • Balance • Body image • Spatial orientation

(continued)

Table 6.4　(continued)

Category	Activity	Purpose
Washcloths	Place • Over, under, next to • On specific body parts Manipulate • Shake • Wring out • Stretch • Crumple • Toss and catch Use • Wash and dry • Cover • Hide • Hold	Orientation to • Being wet all over • Showering Assesses • Grasp and release • Hand and arm strength and endurance • Coordination • Range of motion
Wonderboards	Balance • Seated • Kneeling • Standing Locomotion • Arm pull • Leg pull Directional movement • Seated • Kneeling • Standing Resistance exercises Leg exercises	Orientation to • Equipment for swim instruction • Use of specific body parts in isolation • Resistance of water Assesses • Balance • Arm and leg strength and endurance • Coordination • Endurance

Aquatic Movement Assessment Matrix

Another way of viewing assessment is to look at the different developmental characteristics that can be assessed. You can use the following Aquatic Movement Assessment Matrix with a child to document not only specific functionality but also the degree of developmental attainment. The left-hand column lists the skills you will assess and the specific assessment criteria. The next four columns are for noting the child's degree of mastery. As a child reaches a particular level of competency, enter a date or note progress.

Aquatic Movement Assessment Matrix

Name _____

Assessment date _____

Reassessment date _____

Reassessment date _____

	Not present/ skill just emerging	50% accuracy/ sometimes/ trying	75% accuracy/ usually/ improving	100% accuracy/ always/ skilled
PERCEPTUAL-MOTOR ABILITY				
Balance—big boat, Wonderboard, poly shapes				
Can achieve 4-point balance on boat for 10 sec.				
Can kneel on boat with knees at a 90-degree angle for 10 sec.				
Can sit with legs stretched out straight on boat for 10 sec.				
Can sit on Wonder-board for 10 sec.				
Can kneel on Wonder-board for 10 sec.				
Can stand on spot for 10 sec. in water hip deep.				
Can stand on 1 foot for 10 sec. in water hip deep.				
Can stand on 1 foot for 10 sec. with arms crossed in water hip deep.				
Can stand on 1 foot for 10 sec. with arms crossed and eyes shut in water hip deep.				
Body image—movement exploration, clothing				
Can touch or move arms, legs, trunk, and head.				
Can touch or move facial features.				

(continued)

From Susan J. Grosse, 2007, *Water learning* (Champaign, IL: Human Kinetics).

Aquatic Movement Assessment Matrix *(continued)*

	Not present/ skill just emerging	50% accuracy/ sometimes/ trying	75% accuracy/ usually/ improving	100% accuracy/ always/ skilled
Can touch or move shoulders, hips, elbows, knees, ankles, fingers, and toes.				
Can touch or move hair, belly, back, and knee caps.				
Laterality—poly shapes (footprints and handprints)				
Can take small footprint steps.				
Can cross step.				
Can take large footprint step.				
Can step over a flat obstacle, alternating feet.				
Can alternate footprint and handprint.				
Exhibits presence of dominant hand.				
Directionality—movement exploration				
Can move forward and backward.				
Can move sideward to either side.				
Can turn in circles.				
Can move diagonally.				
Can change level and demonstrate up and down.				
Spatial orientation—noodles, movement exploration				
Can solve movement problems but touches floating objects in the area.				
Can solve movement problems without touching any of the floating objects in the area.				

From Susan J. Grosse, 2007, *Water learning* (Champaign, IL: Human Kinetics).

	Not present/ skill just emerging	50% accuracy/ sometimes/ trying	75% accuracy/ usually/ improving	100% accuracy/ always/ skilled
Can solve movement problems but touches objects on the pool bottom.				
Can solve movement problems but touches floating and sub-merged objects.				
Can solve movement problems without touching floating and submerged objects.				
FITNESS				
Endurance—movement exploration				
Can sustain movement for 5 min.				
Does not express fatigue during activity.				
Strength—big boat				
Can climb onto big boat.				
Can climb out of pool.				
Flexibility—interpretive movement				
Can fully extend arms overhead.				
Can twist trunk to both sides.				
Can lift leg to hip level.				
Can reach diagonally hand to foot on both sides.				
Can look from side to side and up and down.				
Cardiorespiratory—movement problems				
Can speak during active participation.				
Does not appear out of breath.				
Skin color appears normal.				

From Susan J. Grosse, 2007, *Water learning* (Champaign, IL: Human Kinetics).

(continued)

Aquatic Movement Assessment Matrix *(continued)*

	Not present/ skill just emerging	50% accuracy/ sometimes/ trying	75% accuracy/ usually/ improving	100% accuracy/ always/ skilled
MOTOR ABILITY				
Skills—interpretive movement, poly shapes				
Can walk.				
Can run.				
Can hop.				
Can jump.				
Can skip.				
Reflex patterns				
Absence of abnormal patterns.				
Exhibits no movement overflow.				
COGNITION				
Comprehension				
Listens during directions.				
Attempts to follow directions.				
Uses appropriate language.				
Following directions				
Attempts at activity are appropriate.				
Repetition of directions are not necessary.				
Does not attempt to cheat.				
Academics—cone academics, jobs				
Color recognition is appropriate.				
Letter recognition is appropriate.				
Number recognition is appropriate.				
Object recognition and matching are appropriate.				
Math processes are age appropriate.				

From Susan J. Grosse, 2007, *Water learning* (Champaign, IL: Human Kinetics).

	Not present/ skill just emerging	50% accuracy/ sometimes/ trying	75% accuracy/ usually/ improving	100% accuracy/ always/ skilled
Language and reading processes are age appropriate.				
Science and social studies processes are age appropriate.				
PSYCHOSOCIAL SKILL				
Impulse control				
Inappropriate move- ments are absent.				
Aggression is absent.				
Behavior is appropriate.				
Attention span and time on task are appropriate.				
Child is not distractible.				
Interaction with peers is appropriate.				
Participates in isolation play.				
Participates in parallel play.				
Shares.				
Response to environment				
Child is accepting.				
Child is confident.				
Child will submerge.				
Child is fearful.				
Child is fearless.				

Summary Notes

Perceptual-motor ability

_____

_____

Fitness

_____

_____

(continued)

From Susan J. Grosse, 2007, *Water learning* (Champaign, IL: Human Kinetics).

Aquatic Movement Assessment Matrix *(continued)*

Motor ability

____

____

Cognition

____

____

Psychosocial skill

____

____

Assessed by ____________________________

resources

American Psychiatric Association. 1994. *Diagnostic and Statistical Manual of Mental Disorders,* 4th ed. (text revision). Washington, D.C.: American Psychiatric Association.

American Red Cross. 2006. *First Aid/CPR/AED for Schools and the Community.* Yardley, PA: Staywell.

American Red Cross. 1976. *Methods in Adapted Aquatics.* Washington, D.C.: American Red Cross.

Blackmore, C. 2003. Movement is essential to learning. *Journal of Physical Education, Recreation and Dance* 74(9): 22-25, November/December.

Buis, J., and C. Shane. 1989. Movement exploration as a technique for teaching pre-swimming skills to students with developmental delays. In *Best of Practical Pointers,* edited by S. Grosse. Reston, VA: American Alliance for Health, Physical Education, Recreation and Dance.

Cheatum, B., and A. Hammond. 2001. *Physical Activities for Improving Children's Learning and Behavior: A Guide to Sensory Motor Development.* Champaign, IL: Human Kinetics.

Crosser, S. 1994. Making the most of water play. *Young Children* 49(5), 28-32, July.

Curry Lawrence, C., and L. Hackett. 1975. *Water Learning.* Palo Alto, CA: Peek.

Denwiddie, S.A. 1993. Playing in the gutters: Enhancing children's cognitive and social play. *Young Children* 48(6), 70-73, September.

Diem, L. 1982. Early motor stimulation and personal development. *Journal of Physical Education, Recreation and Dance* 53(9): 23-25, November/December.

Gabbei, R., and H. Clemmens. 2005. Creative movement from children's storybooks. *Journal of Physical Education, Recreation and Dance* 76(9): 32-38, November/December.

Grosse, S. 2005. *Aqua Beat.* Milwaukee, WI: Aquatic Consulting and Education Resource Services.

Gulley, S.B. 1982. The relationship of infant stimulation to cognitive development. *Childhood Education* 58(2): 247-248, March/April.

Hengstman, J. 2001. *Movement ABCs.* Champaign, IL: Human Kinetics.

Hurwitz, J. 2004. Research flows to new depths: Aquatic exercise can enhance brain function. *AKWA* 17(2): December/January.

Iverson, B. 1982. Play, creativity, and schools today. *Phi Delta Kappan* 63(7): 693-694, July.

Johnson, E. 1981. Water: Wet and wonderful but not necessarily wild. *Day Care and Early Education* 8(3): 12-14, Spring.

Kaufman, K. 2006. *Inclusive Creative Movement and Dance*. Champaign, IL: Human Kinetics.

Kephart, N. 1966. *The Slow Learner in the Classroom*. Columbus, OH: Merrill.

Langendorfer, S., and L. Bruya. 1995. *Aquatic Readiness: Developing Water Competence in Young Children*. Champaign, IL: Human Kinetics.

Larson, L. 1977. *Foam Geometric Shapes*. New York: Instructor.

Littman, K., and L. Leslie. 1978. *Preschool Recreation Enrichment Program*. Vol. 2. Washington, D.C.: Hawkins.

Melvin, L. 1970. *Adapting Perceptual-Motor Programs for the Aquatic Environment*. Atlanta: Georgia Department of Human Resources.

Needlman, G. 1981. Make holes in the environment and let children see inside. *Children Today* 10(6): 13-14, November/December.

Prupas, A., W. Harvey, and J. Benjamin. 2006. Early intervention aquatics: A program for children with autism and their families. *Journal of Physical Education, Recreation and Dance* 77(2): 46-52, February.

Sayre, N.E. 1995. *Focus on Preschool Aquatics: Child Care Regulations*. Washington, D.C.: ERIC Clearinghouse. ERIC Document Reproduction Service No. ED 381527.

Sible, K.P. 2000. Water, water everywhere. *Young Children* 55(1): 64-66, January.

Stein, J. 2004. Motor development, the brain, and aquatic therapy. *Aquatic Therapy Journal* 6(2): 19-23, July.

Stevens-Smith, D. 2004. Movement and learning: A valuable connection. *Strategies* 18(1): 10-11, September/October.

Stopka, C. 2001. Equipment to enhance an adapted aquatic program, part 1. *Palaestra* 17(1): 36-43, Spring.

Stopka, C. 2001. Equipment to enhance an adapted aquatic program, part 2. *Palaestra* 17(2): 40-43, Summer.

Stopka, C. 2001. Equipment to enhance an adapted aquatic program, part 3. *Palaestra* 17(3): 39-43, Winter.

Toney, H. 1993. Re-appraising nursery water play. *Early Child Development and Care* 163(2): 29-35.

Commercial Resources

Aquam (big boats), 1320 Route 9, Champlain, NY 12919, 1-877-766-5872, www.aquam.com

Aquatic Consulting and Education Resource Services (poly shapes, publications, workshops), 7252 W. Wabash Avenue, Milwaukee, WI 53223, http://my.execpc.com/~grosse.

Aquatics by Sprint (Wonderboards), P.O. Box 3840, San Luis Obispo, CA 93403, 1-800-235-2156; www.sprintaquatics.com

Poly Enterprises (poly shapes), 230 E. Pomona Ave., Monrovia, CA 91016, 626-358-5115, www.polyenterprises.com

Speedo International (steps), 6040 Bandini Blvd., Los Angeles, CA 90040, 1-888-477-3336, www.speedo.com

Wagon Wheel Records (music and water learning recordings), 16812 Pembrook Lane, Huntington Beach, CA 92649, 714-846-8169, www.wagonwheelrecords.net

about the author

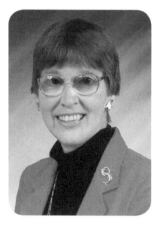

Susan J. Grosse, MS, is the president of Aquatic Consulting & Education Resource Services in Milwaukee. Grosse has more than 45 years of experience in aquatics and education and has published extensively in the areas of aquatics and exceptional education. She is also a sought-after speaker, having presented in Ireland, Egypt, Canada, and across the United States.

Grosse received a 40-year pin from the American Red Cross as a volunteer instructor and instructor trainer. She also received the Mabel Lee and Honor Awards from the American Alliance for Health, Physical Education, Recreation and Dance (AAHPERD) for her contributions to the education profession. The Aquatic Therapy and Rehab Institute presented her with a Tsunami Spirit Award for her work in aquatics with people with disabilities.

Grosse has served as chair of the Aquatic Council for AAHPERD and as president of the American Association for Active Lifestyles and Fitness. She also has been a water safety instructor trainer and a lifeguarding instructor trainer for the American Red Cross. She can't get enough of the water: In her leisure time she enjoys swimming and canoeing as well as reading and listening to music.